Weight Training for Women Over 40

A Complete Guide to Weight Training and
Workout Programs for Building Strength

Carolyn Eldridge

Table of Contents

Introduction

When I was 7 years old, I began competing in track. My first time participating in track and field was awful. I was a clumsy, thin sprinter. I improved as a technical sprinter over time and eventually ran for UCLA in college. At the college level, all students were forced to participate in weightlifting and track practices. At this point, I had gained a lot of knowledge about powerlifting and developed a strong interest in weightlifting. I worked hard to gain additional bulk since I was still much thinner than my colleagues and wanted to be more competitive. I also became weary of the other students making fun of me for being too little and "not curvaceous." Compared to what I was witnessing on the track, I saw benefits in the gym far more quickly. It was really challenging for me to become faster with each session, yet it was quite simple for me to lift more weight at each practice. This encouraged me to continue going to practice and putting more weight on the bar each time. I was aware that gaining muscle bulk would be challenging for me, but I persisted and ultimately succeeded after many years of regular exercise. It was remarkable to be able to lift so much weight while being so little. I wanted to be stronger than the non-athletic males at my gym.

After I got my degree in physiological science, I decided not to follow my first goal of going to graduate school for physical therapy.I decided to get certified as a personal trainer so I could learn how to help people in a more practical way. I still wanted to learn how to treat and prevent injuries, but this was a better way to do that.That was the wisest choice I've ever made! I gained a lot of knowledge, not just about avoiding injuries but also about functional training in general.

Weightlifting has given me a sense of strength and power that I believe all women should aspire to. I wrote this book for that reason. I want to utilize all the information I've learned over the years to guide ladies starting their weightlifting careers in the right direction.

I also want to demonstrate to women that lifting weights is powerful and won't devalue their femininity. In fact, lifting weights makes your body's inherent contours pop even more!

Every woman should consider weightlifting, regardless of age, background, or body type. I'm sure you'll keep going once you start on your quest. The strength and power you acquire will transform your life, and they are genuinely valuable.

8 Benefits of Weight Training

Why should you start lifting weights? Despite appearances, weightlifting has numerous positive effects on one's physical, mental, and emotional wellbeing. There are many physical advantages to weight training besides just increasing your strength, which is what most people expect it to do. These advantages include improving your bone density, metabolic rate, cognitive function, coordination, and stability, as well as your cardiovascular and energy systems. Many of these advantages make you feel powerful physically and psychologically and influence how you approach each day. The specifics and scientific evidence for each of these amazing advantages are provided below.

1. An increase in power You may build the muscular strength required to move heavier things both inside and outside of the gym by lifting weights. If you had powerful muscles, imagine how much simpler duties like carrying in the groceries and scooping up your kids and dogs would be! Strengthening your muscles will also help to support your bone structure and keep you standing straight. 2. Enhanced bone mass Speaking of bones, many women face the danger of aging-related bone deterioration known as osteopenia or osteoporosis. By improving bone density, weightlifting helps keep your bones robust as you age. Your body is forced to create more

bone tissue as a result of exercising the muscles that are connected to your bones, strengthening and increasing the density of your bones. It has two wonderful advantages in one!

3. A faster metabolism Your total muscle mass will increase as a consequence of strength training, and the more muscle you have, the more calories you burn at rest. This is due to the higher calorie expenditure of muscular tissue. When you have greater muscle mass, you will burn more calories even when you're not exercising.

4. Enhanced mental capacity In essence, strength training improves cognitive function. With strength training, your brain must function differently. It must be able to recall your movement patterns, locate your limbs in relation to your body, and pay attention to external inputs. This requires a lot of mental effort, particularly if you are new to weight training. Thus, it's a great method to exercise your brain. Weightlifting releases happy hormones (endorphins) into your system, which not only makes you smarter but also helps to enhance your mood and boost your self-esteem.

5. Better steadiness and coordination Gaining more stability, coordination, and proprioceptive input via weightlifting and coordinated motions (how your brain recognizes where your body and limbs are when performing movements). This helps keep you from falling or having awkward moments.

6. A greater ability of the heart While lifting weights may not appear like cardio, it is when done at an intensity that causes your heart rate to increase. You repeatedly perform the exercises' actions in a rhythmic manner. Also, when you superset workouts—that is, execute activities back-to-back with little to no recovery between them—your heart rate remains elevated. This turns lifting weights into a sort of cardio (and it's far more fun than utilizing cardio machines!)

7. Improved cellular processes As you lift weights, your blood lactate levels, hemoglobin levels, and capillary-to-fiber ratio all rise. These elevations improve blood flow throughout the body, which helps your cells work more effectively. The transport of oxygen and

nutrients to the muscles increases with improved blood flow efficiency, leading to optimum cellular function.

8. Reduction of stress By allowing your body and brain to release any stored emotions, weightlifting reduces stress. Your body uses the hormones created during exercise to balance the stress-inducing hormone cortisol. Moreover, weightlifting helps you develop self-esteem and confidence, both of which help you cope with stress. Therefore, in addition to getting to move some weight to relax and reduce tension, working out releases stress-relieving chemicals that help you feel more confident afterward.

Every woman should consider weightlifting, regardless of age, background, or body type. I'm sure you'll keep going once you start on your quest. The strength and power you acquire will transform your life, and they are genuinely valuable.

Identify Your Goals

It's time for you to choose a goal now that you are aware of some of the fantastic advantages of working out. Establishing goals increases motivation and fulfillment on a personal level. You must choose a goal that is firmly entrenched in your "WHY" in the first place. You place a lot of importance on your WHY. That isn't anything trivial or unimportant. Instead, your WHY is something that you personally link with an emotional response—a powerful internal drive that is unique to you. You will be less likely to achieve your objective if it doesn't have a why behind it. Also, you must desire to accomplish that goal for your own sake and not because someone else has set it for you.

Making sure your objective is SMART, or specific, measurable, achievable, realistic, and time-sensitive, is the next stage. For instance, "I want to lose 10 pounds in two months so that I may engage in more activities on our forthcoming family trip." might be a SMART goal. Three times a week of weightlifting is how I plan to do this. It is extremely definite, quantifiable, and doable to lose 10 pounds in 2 months if you do it within the time span allotted. The fact that this guy can lift weights three times per week is also feasible. The WHY for the SMART goal may be "I want to engage in more activities on vacation because I don't want to be left out of the family photographs or lose out on creating memories as a family." to take it a step further. Given that they chose this goal for themselves rather than having someone else choose it for them, this individual is far more likely to lose the 10 pounds since their WHY has a deep emotional connection to it.

How Frequently Should I Workout?

Your objectives and way of life will actually determine when and how frequently you should exercise. The most essential thing is to establish and adhere to a regimen. Examine your schedule and decide how many days a week you can reasonably devote to working out. Based on your schedule and amount of energy throughout the day, decide if mornings, afternoons, or nights are the ideal times for you to exercise. You could even decide that a different time of day suits you better. As long as you consistently exercise for the number of days you commit to, it won't have an impact on the program's outcomes. The very least you must commit to in order to observe improvements in your body is two days of exercise each week. While it's best to exercise for at least 3 days, some individuals can manage 4 or 5 depending on their objectives and workout style. You may want to think about beginning with fewer days and gradually increasing them as your exercise regimen develops. Aggressiveness and a long start might cause you to have unreasonable expectations of yourself and damage your drive.

Your exercises should be scheduled to last between 30 and 90 minutes, not counting warm-up and cool-down periods. Your weightlifting program's duration will be determined by your goals. If you want to burn fat or lose weight, make circuits of three or four exercises that you do one after the other for a set. Less time will be spent working out, and fewer rest breaks will be required. The emphasis of your workout will be one exercise at a time or supersets with enough rest and recovery periods if you're seeking to gain muscle. This kind of training will need more time and maybe more workouts to exhaust a certain muscle group. The number of days you commit to exercising will also influence how long you spend working out. For instance, 30- to 45-minute intervals would be a reasonable amount of time to help avoid overtraining if you were exercising four or five times each week. (Overtraining occurs when you overtrain and don't give your body enough time to recuperate.) 60 to 90 minutes would be great to optimize benefits if you can only work out 2 or 3 times per week since you are committed to fewer days.

6 Tips to Maintain a Life of Lifting

Beyond only being good for the body, weightlifting has many other advantages. While aesthetics may be what first draws you in or what you learn more about, the other advantages listed at the beginning of this chapter may enrich your life in a variety of different ways. Because of this, you discover that you want to include weightlifting in your daily routine. Finding additional driving forces that keep you linked to a WHY that goes beyond looks is the key to achieving this. Here are some suggestions for finding those additional motivating elements that can help you continue lifting throughout your life.

1. Avoid lifting only for show. When you first start, being attractive is a terrific way to inspire yourself. But what happens as you age? You may not seem the same as you once did when your body begins to alter as you get older. If so, fantastic! But it's possible that your ideal aesthetic appearance won't be sustainably managed. Concentrate on learning a certain exercise that you previously couldn't accomplish or on lifting a certain amount of weight. These kinds of pressing objectives will keep you lifting for a longer period of time than just aesthetic ones.

2. Pay attention to your body. While weightlifting is excellent, it does place a little more pressure on your body, so you should be wise and pay attention to what it is telling you. Be sure to move in ways that your body will like. Also, take a nap when your body tells you to.

3. Schedule time for rest. As was already discussed, there are many things you can do to take better care of your body. Spend some time each day foam rolling and stretching, or learn other self-myofascial release (SMR) techniques. SMR uses a variety of massage methods and instruments to remove knots, or trigger points, from the fascia of your muscles. Furthermore, massages are helpful for your muscles' recovery, as are getting enough water and sleep.

4. Get a personal trainer. You may avoid becoming bored with your routine by working with a personal trainer. To assist you in avoiding injuries and receiving the right amount of recuperation in between exercises, they can also create routines for you. The cost of a personal trainer is justified. The cost of making an investment in your health is never too expensive.

5. Change things up. Changing up your routine prevents boredom. As your confidence in weight training grows, experiment with incorporating other techniques and tools into your workouts, such as kettlebells, TRX (total-body resistance exercise) straps, a ViPR (short for "vitality, performance, and reconditioning"), resistance bands, machines, and cables. Your body and mind will have to work together as you learn to control motions using novel training stimuli.

6. Keep things moving. Motivate yourself to take action each day. Make lifting weights a habit rather than a chore. You can keep what you have by moving a little bit every day, so get moving or you'll lose it!

EQUIPMENT AND ENVIRONMENT

This chapter will focus on the things you should think about when evaluating your training environment and the equipment you have.You may want to work out at home and require information on what you'll need at home to set up your own gym, depending on your objectives and schedule. You could decide to work out at a gym where a trainer can meet you at set times if you think having a trainer and/or a specialized workout area would help you remain motivated. We'll talk about what to expect, how to act, and what to wear so that you feel ready and confident when you go to the gym.Do you understand the distinctions between machines and free weights? We'll examine the tools that will support your program the most and why. We'll examine the factors you should think about while making these choices in order to be safe and have a successful weightlifting regimen.

Exercise at Home vs. the Gym

Felt frightened while lifting weights at a gym? The emotion is natural; there's no need to worry. You will learn all you need from this book, enabling you to approach the weight rack with self-assurance and a training schedule in hand.

There are a few significant distinctions between exercising at home and at a gym. The first is the equipment choice. The gym has a wide range of aerobic and weightlifting machines, which is crucial as you advance in your program and need heavier weights. Dumbbells, kettlebells, barbells, resistance bands, cables, and machines in various sets will be at your disposal. Also, there will be larger weights with safety features at your disposal, including a leg press machine and a weightlifting rack where you may do powerlifting exercises. Because of the safety of the rack, this kind of equipment enables you to lift weights that are considerably heavier than you can at home. Even though it may seem overwhelming to think about everything, having all these alternatives gives you greater flexibility to choose what is best for you and your health. Another thing to keep in mind about the gym is that there are trainers there who can show you how to use the equipment properly and keep an eye on you to make sure you're doing it appropriately.

The gym is another great motivator because going there takes work and physical effort, while sitting at home doesn't.Some individuals discover that they are more likely to stick to their training routines if they arrange their gym time while they do other activities and are not at home getting sidetracked. Also, you are more inclined to push yourself while you are at the gym since you are in a social environment.

Take modest steps if, after reading this book, you still have any trepidation about lifting weights at the gym. Get some weights to get started, then choose a spot in the gym to work out. If your gym offers a studio for classes, using the studio when there are no classes in session gives you a more private workout space. If you're still unable to visit the gym, this book is filled with "home workout hack" advice that will help you maximize your program while you're at home.

The use of a gym has drawbacks. There may be a queue to use the equipment at times, and you may have to wait for someone else to complete using a piece of it before you can use it. Moreover, even though most gyms are quite clean, you can discover that several of the equipment handles and chairs need to be cleaned off in between usage due to constant, uninterrupted use. At home, you never have to wait in line for anything, and everything is always spotless and available for use. But even though a home gym may seem perfect, bear in mind that you'll probably have a smaller selection of equipment at your disposal and that as you advance in your weightlifting program, you'll need to keep buying larger weights. Whatever option you choose, you must figure out how to make the most of your application. The most important thing is that no matter where you are, you make a commitment to yourself and follow through.

What Weight

Free weights and machines are the two main categories of weights to take into account. Any weight that you may utilize unrestrictedly in all planes of motion is referred to as a free weight. Simply put, you have complete control over them since they aren't connected to anything. The benefit of utilizing free weights is that they are the most useful pieces of equipment, allowing you to move in the same manner that you do while going about your regular tasks in real life. Your muscles will grow under various types of stress with the aid of free weights, which is crucial for avoiding injuries and improving mobility in general. Free weights need greater caution as well, since you have total control over them. As a result, if you utilize the weights improperly, nothing will protect you. The machinery is set in place. Just one line of tension and one motion are permitted while pushing or pulling the weight. While safer, this is not practical. In actual life, it's uncommon for your body to travel in a straight line along a single plane. This implies that even while utilizing a machine, you might still put yourself at risk for injury since the machine may not be a good fit for your natural movement patterns and anatomical structure.

Every workout described in the book uses free weights, making it simple to do the exercises in the gym or at home. Free weights also make it possible for the workout measures to stay consistent, which is crucial for monitoring your development. You must always be aware of the weight you are lifting in order to appropriately track your development. The next parts will go through the different free weights that are utilized in this book. The majority of the exercises in this book may be performed with any sort of free weight, so keep that in mind.

DUMBBELLS

Short bars with weights at either end are dumbbells. You may use dumbbells alone or in pairs. You'll be able to exercise each arm separately as a result (called unilateral training). This is an excellent way to ensure that your muscles are balanced and that one arm isn't overcompensating for the other. Dumbbells have the additional advantage of allowing you to hold them closer or further away from your body, depending on what feels comfortable to you, in order to best suit your joints. The dumbbells may also be turned both internally and externally for comfort. Dumbbells are also simpler to drop while executing an exercise if you really must. Never let your weights fall, particularly while switching between workouts. Yet, dropping the weights is safer than continuing to hold on to the dumbbells and running the danger of damage if you don't have a spotter and your muscles are exhausted to failure. Always make sure you are in an open area and that you won't harm anybody if you have to drop the weights.

BARBELLS

Contrarily, barbells feature a longer metal rod with weight disks attached to either end. You may change the weight at either end of certain barbells. Like dumbbells, other barbells have a set weight. Using barbells, you may load up for leg workouts. (Adding extra weight to a movement is known as "loading"). Due to the fact that women frequently have stronger lower bodies than upper bodies, using heavier weights with barbells is simpler because your shoulders and upper back carry the weight rather than just your arms. Also, since you can grab a barbell with both hands, it might sometimes seem simpler to handle. This is because you can better steady yourself while executing pushing and pulling motions. Be mindful that barbells might enable you to compensate by pressing more forcefully with one side than the other. Barbells are also a bit more difficult to move about the house and a little heavier than dumbbells. Barbells are a terrific tool once you learn how to utilize them, particularly for workouts where you want to use more weight. Dumbbells may be used in place of barbells for workouts, but you run the danger of slipping before finishing a set. It is not ideal to have to stop the action at this point and set the dumbbells down before completing the exercise.

ETIQUETTE DU GYM

If you want to keep the gym atmosphere friendly, it's crucial to practice proper gym etiquette. Nobody likes to lift weights with the lady who breaks the rules. Be not that lady. These are some things to remember.

Don't overuse the tools. Everyone is attempting to fit in their exercises despite having a time and equipment crunch. After you've finished your set, let someone else use the apparatus while you relax. To share is to care!

Leave the area tidy. Other kindergarten norms, like sharing, also apply at the gym, like putting the equipment back where it belongs. Reorganize your weights and clean everything, including benches, chairs, balls, handles, and cardio equipment that may have come into contact with your sweat.

Avoid talking on the phone. Nobody wants to let your most recent gossip keep them from exercising. Move your discussion to the lobby. Although texting is OK, you should be aware of how much time you spend perched on a piece of furniture. You may take a two-minute break. Any time after that, you should stop using the device or bench and let someone else use it.

Request a partner to collaborate with. Don't simply take someone else's weights or equipment without asking first. Ask them nicely how many sets they have left if you want to utilize a piece of equipment that they are currently using. After that, you may either wait for them to finish or offer to work alongside them, using the weights or other equipment while they relax.

Maintain proper hygiene. Wear clean gym attire and take the necessary precautions to avoid odor after you begin perspiring by reapplying deodorant or antiperspirant before your exercise. If you can smell yourself, chances are others can too, according to a decent rule of thumb. Furthermore, include a towel so you can wipe down any equipment or yourself that becomes sweaty. When everyone maintains decent hygiene, the gym is much better.

Avoid making things uncomfortable for others. The gym is often crowded with attractive individuals with excellent physiques. They are there to exercise, just as you are, however. Be sociable, but keep in mind that the gym is more or less a workplace and not a nightclub.

Respect the workouts of others. It's OK to take motivation from a fellow participant's or a trainer's exercise. Don't, however, duplicate every exercise move someone else does. You don't know what they're trying to accomplish, and if they're pros, you're stealing their exercise. Going up to the individual when they're free and asking if they would mind helping you create some of your own routines is much nicer. Also, you might ask them to go through the advantages of the activity you were considering replicating.

Clothes and other equipment

To allow for dynamic movements, most ladies go to the gym wearing shorts or leggings. Sweatpants are also OK; however, you could become too hot in them. Select breathable, moisture-wicking bottoms that are made for exercise to avoid pain or, worse, an infection. (For that reason, cotton underwear is also recommended.) Wear a moisture-wicking shirt and a supportive sports bra as well. Depending on your degree of comfort, you may choose a tank top, a short-sleeved shirt, or a long-sleeved shirt. Polyester, nylon, spandex, and cotton are suggested materials for shirts and bottoms.

You should also put on a pair of sports shoes. It would be ideal to use a cross-training sneaker rather than a running shoe or a regular sneaker. To allow for stability and dynamic mobility when weightlifting, the shoe should be supportive and reasonably flat. To choose which brand is ideal for you, it is essential to visit an athletic shop and try on a few different options. Try on your first pair of shoes and do a few dynamic actions like walking, leaping, and squatting, as everyone's feet are unique. To correct any imbalances in your feet, you may also require insoles.

There are a few things you should think about when it comes to extra products. Weighted gloves are helpful for strengthening your grip and preventing calluses on your hands. Together with a few towels to place on shared equipment and a water bottle to keep you hydrated throughout your exercise, it is a good idea to bring these items with you. To prevent the gym floor from becoming cluttered, it is also helpful to carry a little drawstring bag to the gym.

Constructing a Home Gym

I advise getting a set of dumbbells and a barbell to do the exercises in this book if you want to train at home rather than at a gym. Get a dumbbell set with adjustable weight instead of one with a fixed weight so that you only need one set rather than many. In order to make the most of your space, the same logic applies when choosing a barbell: look for one that lets you add and remove weight plates. If you want to store your weights outdoors, it is a good idea to get iron dumbbells and barbells since they withstand severe weather conditions better. The vibrant neoprene weights are available for use inside.

A weight bench might be beneficial for you if you have the room. A foam roller, a stability ball, resistance bands, a medicine ball, ankle weights, booty bands, a yoga mat, and a step are other items to think about getting. You can buy a set of resistance bands that let you swap out the grips to create different levels of resistance. (Similar to how dumbbells and barbells were suggested above, this is helpful for saving space.) Choose your items depending on what you believe is acceptable for your level of fitness. The equipment is all really practical and will enhance your at-home weightlifting experience. All of this equipment is available for online purchase, which is wonderful since it allows for doorstep delivery. You may want to browse online for gym storage suggestions to keep your equipment arranged and out of the way.

Set up your training area in a place with enough light and, if possible, a mirror so you can keep an eye on your form as you move.You don't want to accidently walk on anything or knock something over; therefore, you need enough free space for dynamic motions. Carpet is helpful since it provides additional cushioning for floor workouts and helps to muffle sounds when setting the weights down. But, bear in mind that a carpet will be less stable (which will make motions more difficult) and that a carpet is more difficult to remove perspiration from. For your home gym, I would suggest installing a rubber surface that is simple to keep clean. This kind of floor is simple to maintain, solid, and has a little give to it to help absorb the impact of more erratic motions. While wooden floors are OK, it is advised that you place something in between the floor and the weights to prevent scuffs.

Consider installing a sound system in your home gym if you want to listen to music while you exercise. Having a water supply nearby where you can rehydrate throughout your exercises may also be a smart idea. To keep the gym at the right temperature while working out, you might also need to use a fan or a portable heater. All things considered, the price of a home gym depends on the quantity of equipment you need and the amount of usable space you desire. You may get started with a modest $50 investment for a few weights. A whole set of free weights may set you back $500. You may wish to get some cardio equipment for your home gym as you advance. Your final cost can be closer to $2,000 as a result. Start modestly with your first purchase, and as your enthusiasm for weightlifting builds, add additional equipment.

GLUTES AND HAMSTRINGS

The muscles in your buttocks, known as the glutes, maintain your pelvis when you undertake activities like walking and standing. They also aid in actions like turning the thigh outward. The gluteus maximus, gluteus medius, and gluteus minimus are the muscles that make up this group.

The muscles that run down the backs of your thighs are called hamstrings. The semimembranosus, semitendinosus, and biceps femoris muscles make up this group. This muscle group is in charge of knee flexion and hip extension (bending your knee). Your hamstrings are used for actions like stepping up and jogging. It's vital to remember that your core is made up of many muscular groups, including your hamstrings and glutes. Contrary to popular belief, your core is not just made up of your abdominal muscles. Each muscle that helps your upper and lower halves move in unison is considered to be part of your core. You need to properly prepare these muscles since you utilize them for everyday tasks in order to prevent injury or strain. Preparing them for exercise and stretching them afterward requires additional time.

Individuals often believe that they need to stretch their hamstrings more because they are "tight," but for the majority of people, this is not the case. Long-term seated individuals develop shortening in their gluteal, hip, and lower back muscles. During extended sitting, the muscle fibers stay short or constricted, which is referred to as shortness. The hamstrings are lengthened as a consequence of the pelvis rotating in this manner. The sensation of tightness that most people relate to is really that of tautness since the muscle has reached its maximum length and no longer has space to move. Instead of overstretching the hamstrings to avoid this, think about doing exercises like the pretzel stretch in this chapter that will extend the hips and activate the glutes.

WARM-UP

STRAIGHT-LEG KICK

Since they resemble the fictitious figure when executed, straight-leg kicks are sometimes referred to as Frankenstein or monster kicks. It's a fantastic exercise for warming up the core and actively extending the hamstrings.

1. Place your feet hip-width apart and stand.2. Kick your right leg into the air and try to touch your toes with your left hand while stepping forward with your left leg.
3. Return to the beginning position, and then step forward with your right leg, kicking your left leg into the air, and reaching for your toes with your right hand.
4. Continue this exercise by going forward and kicking your legs alternately in front of you until you feel warmed up. By doing this exercise, you should seem and feel like Frankenstein's monster.

WARM-UP

BEST STRETCH IN THE WORLD

This stretch is excellent for extending the hip joint's range of motion, improving mobility, and giving the hamstrings a dynamic stretch. It also warms up your core and upper body. Because it stretches so many different muscle groups at once, it is known as the World's Biggest Stretch.

1. Place your feet hip-width apart and stand. Reach down to the ground with your hands while pivoting from your hips. To experience a wonderful stretch in your hamstrings, try to touch the ground without bending your knees.
2. After placing your hands' palms on the floor, move your hands

forward until you are in the push-up posture. Bend your knees just a little to help you reach if you are unable to put your hands on the ground. Your shoulders and hips have to be in line.

3. Step forward with your left foot and plant it outside of your left hand. Lift your left hand into the air while you press your right hand into the ground. Next, expand your chest toward your left side by rotating through your thoracic spine. Your eyes should follow your hand.

4. Return your foot to the push-up starting position after bringing your hand back to the floor.

5. Step forward with your right foot, putting it on the floor next to your right hand, then rotate to the other side.

6. Go back into the push-up position. As you walk back to a standing posture, elevate your hips, keep your legs straight, and try to keep your heels down as you move your hands back toward your feet.

EXERCISE

DEADLIFT

Both the upper body and lower body muscles are used in this intricate dance. Furthermore, it is excellent for neurological coordination and core development.

1. Hold dumbbells or a barbell in your hands while you stand with your feet hip-width apart and your toes pointing forward.

2. Hinge from your hips and push your buttocks back as though you're attempting to make them contact a wall that doesn't exist. To work the hamstrings, keep your knees supple but do not bend them. When you reach and bring the weights toward your shins, maintain a flat back and press your shoulder blades together to activate the upper back muscles. Avoid rounding or overextending your back.

3. After you've reached the lowest point in your range of motion

without arching your back, squeeze your glutes to propel your hips forward and bring you back to a standing posture.

Raise Caution: You should only feel this workout in your glutes and hamstrings. If you encounter any lower back discomfort, stop lifting weights and concentrate only on your hip-hinging technique. Making It Simpler Feel free to experiment with where you place your feet. For the deadlift's final posture, you may require a wider (or narrower) stance to prevent your spine from rounding. To put your body in the best posture, you may also need to turn your feet slightly outward so that your toes point out.

EXERCISE

SINGLE-LEG ROMANIAN DEADLIFT

Worked additional muscles: rear, core
This exercise targets the same muscle group as the deadlift but adds complexity by testing your balance. Also, it aids in balancing out any right-to-left asymmetries.

1. Hold a dumbbell or barbell in front of you with both hands, elbows straight, and the weight close to your body while standing with your feet hip-width apart. (Almost like you intend to scratch your shins on the way down with the weight.)

2. Hinge from your hips and raise one foot off the ground, keeping your elbows straight. When you lower your torso and shift the weight toward your shins, letting your leg come up behind you, hinge from your hips. While you kick your leg back, visualize kicking your heel to the sky and flexing your toes toward your shin. (You want your foot and shoulders to swing together, like a pendulum.) Try not to lower the weight to the ground. Once you see a rounding of your spine, stop.

3. Go back to the upright posture you started with. If necessary, you

may put your foot down in between repetitions to get your balance back.

4. Continue on the other leg.

Raise Caution: Avoid opening up at the hips by keeping your back straight and your hips parallel to the ground. Throughout this exercise, you should really feel your hamstrings and glutes working. If you have any back pain, stop using the weights and make form corrections.

Making It Simpler While you are between repetitions, tap your foot on the floor.

Home Exercise Tip: When you do the action without any weight, place a broomstick on your back and try to keep it in touch with your neck, midback, and buttocks. You will gain knowledge about the appropriate spinal alignment via this.

EXERCISE
Glottic Bridge

Exercise Worked More Muscles: Core

This workout is excellent for strengthening and conditioning your hamstrings and glutes. Moreover, it is simpler to master than deadlifts.

1. Lie on your back with your toes pointed forward and your feet hip-width apart on the floor.

2. Hold a dumbbell or barbell in place on your hips, slightly behind your hipbones.

3. Keep your head and shoulders down and relaxed while driving out of your heels and tightening your glutes to raise your hips off the ground. Hold for two seconds at the top of the bridge.

4. Put your hips back on the floor.

Raise Caution: To begin this action, engage your glutes rather than your lower back. Make sure your knees track over your ankles as you complete this exercise. Do not allow them to fall out or collapse in.

Make It Difficult: To execute barbell hip thrusters, use a weight bench or a plyo box. With your feet hip-width apart and your toes pointed forward, sit so that your shoulder blades rest on the bench. Using a pad, position the bar across your hips. Squeeze your glutes at the peak as you raise your hips off the ground. During the action, keep your shoulders firmly planted on the bench and your head and neck in a relaxed position. To move as a single unit, bring your hips back down and move in sync with your shoulders.

EXERCISE
SINGLE-LEG GLUTE BRIDGE EXERCISE

Other muscules that worked: hip flexors, core

In comparison to a typical Glute Bridge, this progression is more challenging. Compared to doing the action with both legs, the single-leg aspect of this exercise forces you to use more of your core and glutes.

1. Lie on your back with your toes pointed forward and your feet hip-width apart on the floor.
2. Hold a dumbbell or barbell in place on your hips, slightly behind your hipbones.
3. Raise your foot one foot up into the air. To raise your hips into a bridge, tighten the glutes of the leg that is on the floor and push with the heel that is firmly planted. Before bringing your hips back down to the ground, hold for approximately 2 seconds.
4. You may alternate legs or complete all the reps on one leg.
Raise Cautiously: During the exercise, make sure your knee stays above your ankle. Keep your back from arching excessively at the

bridge's apex. Do not use your lower back; instead, utilize your glutes to power the action.

Making It Simpler By pushing your hips less high throughout the workout, you may decrease their range of motion. If necessary, forego the weights and carry out this motion using your own body weight.

Increase Difficulty: Employ a heavier weight. During each repetition, you may also move the lifted leg a few inches to the side before bringing it back to the middle. Your core stability will be put to the test even more by this.

EXERCISE
STEP-UP

EXTRA MUSCULES WORKED: Core, Quads, and Hip Flexors

This exercise is excellent for building hamstring and gluteal strength as well as improving balance and stability. It will also make it easier for you to climb and descend staircases.

1. Locate a sturdy step, stool, chair, or box to stand on. Depending on your height and degree of expertise, the surface should be somewhere between 6 and 18 inches from the ground.
2. If you are using dumbbells, place one at your chest and the other at your sides. Put a barbell behind your neck, resting on your shoulders, if you have one.
3. Place your right foot on the chair or box as you stand in front of it.
4. Bring your left leg up until your left knee is at hip height in front of you and drive up through your right leg to stand. After the action has reached its full range, squeeze your right glute.
5. Reverse the motion and put both feet back down on the ground.
6. You may either repeat this movement on the right leg and then switch to the left, or you can swap legs every time.
Lift Safely: While you do step-ups, pay attention to your knee.

During the action, your knee should remain level with your ankle (i.e., not cave in or out). Also, when you step up, maintain your knee behind your toes, and as you step down, do your best to prevent your knee from going too far beyond your toes. Softly touch down, and make sure there are no obstacles in your way for you to trip over as you descend.

Make It Difficult: Each step-up should be performed in a continuous motion without pause. Your equilibrium will be put to the test.

Try exploring around your home for alternative solid surfaces, such as stairs, your patio, or even a sturdy step stool, if you are having problems locating a stable chair for your Step-Ups.

EXERCISE
A LATERAL STEP-UP

Extra muscules worked: core, quads, and hip flexors

Compared to prior step-ups, this exercise will put greater strain on your inner and outer thigh muscles while also encouraging excellent glute activation.

1. Locate a sturdy step, stool, chair, or box to stand on. Depending on your height and degree of expertise, the surface should be somewhere between 6 and 18 inches from the ground.
2. If you are using dumbbells, place one at your chest and the other at your sides. Put a barbell behind your neck, resting on your shoulders, if you have one.
3. Place the box, chair, or step next to you so that it is on your left side.
4.While keeping the box or step to your left, step laterally with your left foot onto it. While you do this, push your right leg up to hip

height with your knee bent at a 90-degree angle. At the peak, squeeze your glutes.

5. Repeat the motion after stepping down and entirely removing your foot from the step or box. Before repeating on the other side, complete all the repetitions on this side.

Lift Safely: While you do step-ups, pay attention to your knee. During the action, your knee should remain level with your ankle (i.e., not cave in or out). Also, when you step up, maintain your knee behind your toes, and as you step down, do your best to prevent your knee from going too far beyond your toes. Softly touch down, and make sure there are no obstacles in your way for you to trip over as you descend.

Make It Difficult: Each step-up should be performed in a continuous motion without pause. Your equilibrium will be put to the test.

Try checking around your home for alternative solid surfaces, such as stairs, your patio, or even a sturdy step stool, if you are having problems locating a stable chair for your step-ups.

STRETCH
PRETZEL STRETCH

Without overstretching the hamstrings, this stretch is ideal for extending the gluteal muscles.

1. Sit with your legs crossed on the ground.
2. Set your left foot on your right knee's outside.
3. Holding your left knee in the crease of your right elbow, extend your right arm. Pulling your left knee into your chest will cause your left glute to stretch while you sit up as straight as you can.
4. Keep the stretch in place and then repeat on the other side.

STRETCH

RESTRICTED TOE TOUCH

Your hamstrings are the focus of this stretch, which makes it crucial.
1. Sit on the ground with your legs straight and your toes pointed forward.
2. Try to touch your toes by extending both arms straight in front of you. Try reaching for your ankles or shins if you can't reach your toes.
3. To maximize the stretch in your hamstrings, keep your knees as straight as you can and bend your toes toward your shins.
4. Continue to stretch.

CALVES AND QUADRICEPS

The phrase "quads" is a shortened form for the quadriceps, a group of muscles at the front of the thigh. The rectus femoris, vastus medialis, vastus lateralis, and vastus intermedius are all parts of this muscle group. The quads' primary function is to extend or straighten the knee. Since it spans the knee and the hip, the rectus femoris is a special muscle. Only the quads' other muscle groups cross the knee joint. Hence, the rectus femoris also aids in hip flexion. You can walk, run, leap, and sit while using these muscles in conjunction with one another. Those who spend most of their days sitting tend to keep this muscle group in high tension. The cause of this is that sitting causes your quadriceps to constantly contract, which drags your pelvic bone forward and causes lower back discomfort as well. Before indulging in explosive sports like running, leaping, and riding, it's a good idea to warm up the quads. Moreover, it's crucial to stretch your quadriceps often if you spend a lot of time sitting during the day.

The muscles on the rear of the lower leg are known as the calves. The gastrocnemius and soleus are two of these muscles. Collectively, they are in charge of flexing, pointing, and rotating the foot inside and outward. The calves are often tight because they have to work so hard to maintain your balance and posture when standing or walking; as a result, they should be stretched frequently to release tension. They are particularly active while performing explosive motions like sprinting and leaping. It is also advised to foam roll and stretch your calves after wearing heels as an additional self-care activity since they are also vulnerable to excess strain if you wear heels often.

Prior to Lifting:
When doing the moves in this chapter, keep your core tight. To ensure proper form, you may also practice each of these moves in front of a mirror or on videotape.

WARM UP
BUTTON KICKER

This is a great dynamic warm-up that stretches the quadriceps by letting them relax, which happens when the hamstrings quickly bend the knees. Based on the reciprocal inhibition principle, which states that one muscle group cannot be active when the opposite or opposing muscle group is in use, this is what is happening.

1. Stand with your feet hip-width apart and lay your hands on your bottom with the palms facing outward.
2. Kick one foot up until your heel softly strikes the palm of your hand. Repeat on the other side after putting your foot back on the ground.
3. The motion may be carried out while stationary or while going forward.

EXERCISE
GOBLET SQUAT

Other muscles worked include the core, glutes, and hamstrings. Goblet squats are a wonderful exercise to improve your squat technique. As you squat, the balancing effect of the front-loaded weight prevents your body from moving too far forward. This is a result of the weight forcing your hips to recline. You'll better grasp how the movement should feel if you imagine it as sitting down and standing up, as you would if you were to sit on a chair.

1. Hold a dumbbell in front of your chest while standing with your feet hip-width apart and toes pointing forward.
2. As you bend your knees and lower yourself into a squat posture, push your hips back and visualize sitting down on a chair.
3. Stop when your knees and hips are at a 90-degree angle at the bottom of the squat.

4. When you're ready to rise up again, force your feet into the floor and push yourself up to stand, clenching your glutes at the top. Raise Caution: During the exercise, maintain a straight back, a raised chest, and equal weight distribution in the centers of your feet. Maintain your knees by moving behind your toes while maintaining the same line of motion as your toes. This is done to safeguard your knees and prevent any harm or discomfort. Also, it guarantees that your glutes are being used correctly. You may experiment with widening or narrowing your stance or turning your feet slightly outward. To squat without your spine curving at the bottom, choose the foot posture that is best for your body type. Reduce your range of motion and stop squatting as low if your back starts to hurt. Making It Simpler When you become acclimated to the squatting position, position a chair behind you on which you may sit. Just your legs and your arms, which are used to support the weight, should feel anything throughout this workout. Put the weight down and practice squatting with only your body weight if your lower back starts to hurt.

Home Exercise Tip: Use your imagination and use whatever object you have around the house as a weight, such as a handbag, your infant, a gallon of water, a backpack, a flower pot, heavy books, or pet food.

EXERCISE
FORWARD LUNGE

Which also works the glutes and hamstrings.

Because of its resemblance to walking in terms of movement pattern, this workout is a useful approach to toning your calves and quads. Also, lunges assist in unilateral leg exercise (one leg at a time). Your bilateral workouts (squats and deadlifts) will get stronger as a result of developing unilateral strength.

1. Achieve a hip-width distance between your feet while standing upright. With your back erect and your shoulder blades tightly pressed together, hold dumbbells in both hands at your sides. Put a barbell over your upper back and along your shoulders if you're using one.
2. Take a big stride forward while bending both legs at the knees. Your rear knee ought to be barely off the floor.
3. To take a stride back and go back to the beginning position, drive out of your front heel. On the other side, repeat
Lift Cautiously: When you lunge forward, make sure your front knee remains in front of your front toes. The path of your ankle and foot should be followed by your front knee as well. While you complete the exercise, keep your chest up and your back straight.
To make it simpler, practice your lunges while stationary and without any weight. While you practice the technique, you may also lean against a wall or grip a stick for balance.
Make It Difficult: Instead of going back to the beginning position, do walking lunges by stepping forward. Bring your rear leg straight through into another forward lunge to make the exercise extra tough by walking continuously throughout it without stopping in the middle of the action.

EXERCISE
LATERAL LUNGE

Glutes, Hamstrings, and Other Muscles Worked

To simulate real-life motions, workouts must be carried out in a variety of planes of motion. While being comparable to the forward lunge, this exercise provides for diverse muscle activation since it is performed in the frontal plane (going side to side). Your inner thighs and outer glute muscles will get greater exercise.

1. Stand with your toes pointed forward and your feet hip-width apart. With your back erect and your shoulder blades tightly pressed together, hold dumbbells at your sides in both hands. Put a barbell over your upper back and along your shoulders if you're using one.

2. Step out to the right and plant your right foot with the toes pointed ahead without rotating your body. When you bring your hips back and down as if you were sitting in a chair, bend your right knee to a 90-degree angle. When you do this, keep your left leg straight and your toes pointing forward.

3. Lift off the ground with your right foot, distributing your weight evenly over your midfoot, and then step back to the beginning position.

4. Continue on the left.

Lift Safely: While you carry out this exercise, maintain a flat back and a high chest. While you lunge, make sure your knee is traveling over your ankle and behind your toes. As you walk to the side, your foot should be straight or slightly turned out, and your shoulders should be square. (Prevent bending your spine in the direction of your lunge.) During the action, you should maintain alignment in your hips, knees, and ankles.

Making It Simpler Exercise without using any weights After you get the hang of the action, you may additionally balance yourself using a stick or a wall. The exercise may be made simpler by adjusting your lunge depth so that you are not lunging as low.

Make It Difficult: Alternately, you may do lateral lunges while walking. To advance with this exercise, you may also add more weight.

EXERCISE
BULGARIAN SPLIT SQUAT

Glutes and hams are additional muscle worked.

Simply put, this exercise is merely another name for an elevated in-place lunge. (The Bulgarian weightlifting system served as the inspiration for the name.) Your calves will be somewhat more worked since the elevation makes it more difficult to maintain balance. To keep your legs balanced in terms of muscle and strength, it also helps each leg get stronger on its own.

1. Face forward and place your feet hip-width apart in front of a chair or box. Across your shoulders and across your back, place a barbell. If using dumbbells, hold one in each hand in front of your chest or at your sides.
2. Gently take up a split stance by placing one foot on the chair behind you. Depending on which position gives you greater stability, the foot on the chair may either be flat and facing down or the toes can be tucked under.
3. Kneel to the floor and do a lunge. A few inches should separate your back knee from the ground. At the bottom of the action, both knees need to be at almost 90 degrees.
4.Return to the beginning posture by planting the heel of your front leg into the ground.
5. Continue on the other side.
Lifting safely requires maintaining a straight back and an elevated chest. Also, maintain a tracking alignment with your ankle and foot, with your front knee behind your front toes. In case you lose your equilibrium, make sure the space around you is free of obstructions. Adjust your feet and chair depth if you have pain in your knees while executing this action. If you don't feel that you have the stability or strength to do so, you don't have to bend all the way to a 90-degree angle.

Making It Simpler A lower-lying chair or surface should be used. The difficulty of the workout will increase with the height of the chair. Use no weight for this exercise to further regress.

EXERCISE
SUITCASE SQUAT EXERCISE MUSCLES

AdditionalGlutes, hamstrings, and core

Similarly to how you move while picking up your bags or your goods from the floor, this is another practical action. It teaches your body how to move a weight away from your center of mass, as with the goblet squats, and toward the ground.

1. Achieve a hip-width distance between your feet while standing upright. On each side of your feet, the dumbbells need to be lying on the ground.
2. Kneel down and pick up the dumbbells from the floor. While you squat, maintain a straight back, a raised chest, and tight shoulder blades. Push your feet forward and stand up while gripping the dumbbells.
3. Squat back down to a roughly 90-degree angle, holding the dumbbells close to your body and at the sides of your knees. While you carry the burden, your weight should be equally distributed between and in the centers of your feet.
4. While holding the dumbbells, squeeze your glutes and tuck your hips to bring yourself back to an upright posture.
5.When you're done with the required number of reps for this exercise, bend down gently to put the dumbbells back on the floor.

Raise Cautiously: While you carry out this motion, be careful to keep your knees behind your toes and your ankles tracking with each other. Adjust the location of your feet and set the weights down if your lower back hurts. Reduce the depth at which you are crouching. Observe your first and final reps carefully. People most often hurt themselves during the first or final rep of a loaded exercise, which involves taking up and setting down weights.

Make It Difficult: Use only one dumbbell to complete the exercise. In order to counterbalance the effects of the dumbbell just pulling down one side of your body, this will cause your core to contract more.

Home Exercise Tip: The next time you go shopping or on vacation, do this at home with your baggage or groceries.

EXERCISE
SINGLE-LEG GOBLET SQUAT EXERCISE.

Biceps, the core, the glutes, and the hamstrings are all worked during the

This exercise is an altered pistol squat. It is excellent for strengthening your unilateral (single-side) muscles and for testing your balance. This exercise is a development of the goblet squat, which develops strength in the bilateral (both sides) muscles.

1. Place your feet hip-width apart as you stand in front of a chair or box. Holding a barbell across your upper back along your shoulders or a dumbbell in front of your chest with both hands is an alternative.
2. Carefully lower yourself to the chair by lifting one foot into the air. Either lift your foot and bend your knee to elevate your leg, or move your whole leg forward without bending your knee. Whatever way is simpler, use it.
3. With the second leg, get out of the chair while keeping the same foot lifted.
4. Before moving on to the next repeat, you may put your foot down on the ground to reestablish stability.
5. Continue with the other leg.

Lifting Safely: When you crouch down to the chair, be cautious to keep your movement under control. Don't just collapse upon the chair. As you squat and stand up, maintain your foot's forward-pointing position and keep your knees behind your toes and tracking with your ankle.

Making It Simpler To make it simpler to stand up, choose a chair that is higher or pile a book on it. A weightless version of this workout is also an option. Until you develop the strength to stand up on one leg, you may also rise up with both legs and sit down on one. Use a shorter chair to make it harder: You may make this harder by using a shorter chair. You may also perform pistol squats with the weight while doing them without the chair.

EXERCISE
CURTSY LUNGE

Additional Muscles Worked: Hamstrings And Glutes

Another exercise that uses a different plane of motion to train your muscles is this one. Rotational motions are those that include twisting and are carried out in the transverse plane. This exercise strengthens the vastus medialis oblique, a muscle in your thighs that you don't use as much as you should.Women's knee injuries may be decreased by strengthening this muscle, particularly for athletes who compete in sports like soccer, basketball, and tennis that require cutting motions.

1. Achieve a hip-width distance between your feet while standing upright. Squeeze your shoulder blades together while keeping your neck relaxed while you hold dumbbells at your sides. Hold the barbell over your upper back and along your shoulders if you're using one.
2. While lowering yourself into a lunge, place one foot behind the other. You need to feel as if you are bowing to the English Queen.

3. Aim to have your hips at the bottom of your lunge with both of your knees at a 90-degree angle.
4. Put your rear foot back in its original position. On the other side, repeat

Raise Caution: During the action, maintain proper alignment in your hips, knees, and ankles. As you lunge, your front knee should follow your ankle and toes without going beyond them, and your shoulders should stay square and pointed forward. Your hips and back shouldn't rotate while you carry out this action. Maintain a straight back throughout.
Making It Simpler To learn the lunge, perform it while keeping your feet in the curtsy posture. While you practice the action, you could grip onto something to support part of your weight.

STRETCH
STANDING CALF STRETCH

Do this standing stretch to ease the tension in your calves and stop them from cramping after your workout. This will give you time to calm down from the exercises you just did.

1. Flex your front toes upward while standing with one foot flat on the ground in front of the other.
2. Lean forward and grasp the front of your feet. Try to maintain the straightest possible knees.
3. Lift your toes up toward your shin until your calf muscles start to tighten. Also, it's okay if your hamstrings feel stretched.
4. Continue on the other side.

STRETCH
STANDING QUAD STRETCH

Women often have a huge set of muscles called the quadriceps that are particularly active. Stretching is crucial after a leg exercise. You can do this simple stretch anywhere.

1. Place your feet hip-width apart and stand.
2. Bend your right knee such that it rises off the ground and goes in the direction of your buttocks.
3. With your right hand, grasp your right ankle. When you feel a stretch in your right quad, pull your foot toward your butt.
4. Gently let go of the foot and place it back on the ground.
5. Continue on the other side.

CHEST

A layer of muscles that begin in your décolletage and extend beneath your breasts make up the chest. The pectoralis major and minor make up this substantial muscle group. You may have heard individuals call their chests "pecs" for this reason.

If your only goal is to look better, you can naturally lift your breasts by working your chest muscles.Some women worry that chest exercises will make their chests smaller because they turn breast tissue into muscle. However, this is not true.Your overall weightlifting is causing you to lose weight, which may result in a decrease in your breast size. If you lose weight just through exercise, the same result may still occur. Since everyone has unique DNA, it is impossible to predict where and when your body will lose weight. Spot training is not allowed, which means you cannot target a certain muscle group in an effort to reduce body fat there. I hope that dispelling any doubts you may have regarding chest training will assist. The advantages of increasing strength outweigh the dangers of going down a cup size as a result of weight reduction in general. As a side note, you may need to take extra care while exercising your chest if you've undergone breast augmentation. You may need to restrict your range of motion or utilize lesser weights. This is a consequence of any scar tissue left behind after the augmentation, if any. Also, it prevents your breasts' look from being harmed by the implants changing. Ask your surgeon for advice on the finest procedures and suggestions.

Prior to Lifting:
When doing the moves in this chapter, keep your core tight. To ensure proper form, you may also practice each of these moves in front of a mirror or on videotape.

WORM-UP
PLANK SCAPTION

Scaptions are an excellent exercise to improve the motion of your shoulder blades. Make sure your shoulder blade muscles are fully warmed since they are crucial to pushing and pulling exercises, particularly in connection with chest motions.

1. To begin, stand in a push-up stance with your arms outstretched, wrists stacked beneath your shoulders, and toes spread apart on the floor. From your heels to your head, draw a single, lengthy line.
2. Pull your shoulder blades toward your spine while keeping your elbows locked and your arms straight (retraction).
3. Maintaining the same posture, pull your shoulder blades closer to your shoulders, away from your spine, and away from each other (protraction). By doing the forward and backward movements over and over again, you can get better at pulling your shoulders in and then out.
4. Aim to move your shoulder blades as much as you can without moving your neck. You may also do this motion while standing up and leaning against a wall.

EXERCISE
DUMBBELL FLOOR PRESS EXERCISE

A basic pushing motion is being used here. It works both of your pectoral muscles, and by utilizing dumbbells rather than a barbell, you can focus on developing your arm strength separately. If you've had a breast augmentation, this exercise is also advised over a conventional bench press (done on a flat bench with a barbell).

1. Lie flat on your back on the floor with your feet hip-width apart and your knees bent. So that you can readily reach the dumbbells,

place them close to your hands at your sides.

2. Lift the weights above you so that they are squarely over your chest while keeping your arms straight and your elbows locked. Your hands should be facing out, and the dumbbells should be horizontal to each other with your thumbs facing each other.

3. While simultaneously bending your elbows to 90 degrees and spreading them apart, lower the dumbbells to your chest. As your elbows reach the ground, stop.

4. Push the weights back up to the starting position by bringing your elbows close together.

Raise Caution: When you complete this exercise, keep your rib cage down and your lower back flat on the floor. Keep your back straight; this will keep your core engaged. Keep your elbows from locking at the peak of the action.

Make It Harder: To make this exercise a bit more challenging, elevate both of your feet into the air so that you are standing on top of a table, knees over hips, and calves parallel to the floor. More core stability will be necessary for this. Moreover, you can only push one dumbbell at a time. To offset the rotating force caused by the imbalanced weight distribution, extra stability will be necessary.

Home Exercise Tip: Push-ups are a great way to build chest muscle without the use of weights. Push-ups may be made simpler by bending at the knees or by placing your hands on a bench or other raised surface.

EXERCISE
DUMBBELL CHEST FLY

Additional muscles used: triceps

Compared to the dumbbell floor press, this exercise somewhat differs in how it targets the chest. The parts of your chest that might make your breasts look closer together will get stronger as a result. The primary goal of this workout is to increase strength, but the added cosmetic advantages are welcome. It's also important to note that if you've undergone breast augmentation, this chest workout will be more accommodating than the barbell floor press.

1. Sit on the floor with your feet hip-width apart and your knees bent. To make it simple for you to pick up the dumbbells, they should be placed near your hands and at your sides.
2. With your arms extended, pick up the weights and place them over your chest with your palms facing each other and your thumbs pointing in the direction of your face.
3. Extend your arms out in front of you, elbows slightly bent, as if you're about to hug a tree or grasp a huge beach ball.
4. Drop the weights until your elbows are at chest height and stop. Only a few inches will separate this from the ground. Keep the weights off the ground at all times.
5. Squeeze your elbows together to bring your arms back to the beginning position.

Lift Safely: While you carry out this exercise, keep your lower back flat on the floor. Avoid hunching your back; this will keep your core engaged. On the way down, avoid reaching out with your arms. When your chest reaches a comfortable stretch, stop. While you do this action, keep the weights directly in front of your chest. They shouldn't hang down by your belly button or hang up by your neck or head.

Make It Difficult: To get greater core activation, do the exercise with your feet off the ground, knees over hips, and calves parallel to the floor. To make it tougher, you may also move only one dumbbell at a time or switch sides rather than moving the weights simultaneously.

EXERCISE
WIDE-GRIP BARBELL CHEST PRESSES

Additional Muscles. Triceps

This press is different from the other chest exercises in this chapter because it uses a wide grip to work a different part of the chest. Your muscles will remain balanced and at their ideal pressing strength thanks to it.

1. Sit on the floor with your feet hip-width apart and your knees bent. When you lay down, the barbell should be in your hands.

2. Hold the barbell with broad hands immediately over your chest; try to get your pinkies as near as possible to the weighted ends of the barbell.

3. Drop the bar toward your chest while maintaining its position just above your midsection. As your elbows reach the ground, halt.

4. In order to press the bar back up, squeeze your elbows together. Raise Caution: While you push the weight, maintain a flat lower back on the floor. Avoid hunching your back. While you push, maintain straight wrists and a low chest. After the exercise is complete, slowly roll up to a sitting posture facing forward while holding the bar in your hands. Never try to shove the bar out to the side or behind you. It would be nice if you had a spotter nearby to help remove the barbell from your grasp. If you've undergone breast augmentation, you may need to apply less force or refrain from this action.

Make It Difficult: To get greater core activation, do the exercise with your feet off the ground, knees over hips, and calves parallel to the floor.

Home Exercise Tip: Do push-ups with your hands wider than shoulder-width apart if you don't have a barbell. 2 inches should separate your hands from the shoulder joint. By placing your hands on a bench or counter top, you may also do a raised, wide push-up. If you've undergone breast augmentation and want to strengthen your chest, this is a terrific option.

STRETCH
WALL STRETCH

The chest muscles are often very tight because of things like texting, typing, and driving.Stretching after working out is important to help the muscle get back to its original length, since working out makes this muscle group even tighter.This wall stretch should also be done after spending a lot of time at a computer or behind the wheel of a vehicle. Shoulder impingements and restricted shoulder motion may result from a tight chest.

1. Place the doorframe on your right side as you stand in a doorway. Put your right foot behind you and your left foot slightly in front of you.
2. Align your elbow so that it forms a 90-degree angle with your shoulder and place your right hand on the doorframe.
3. Until you feel a stretch in your chest, push your torso forward while simultaneously pressing your arm against the doorframe. While you do this, try to avoid arching your back.
4. Continue on the other side.

ABOVE BACK

The trapezius and rhomboids are two of the main muscle groups that make up the upper back. Your skull's base all the way up to the center of your spine is where the trapezius muscles, sometimes known as "traps," are located. The upper, middle, and lower traps are in charge of different movements, like raising and lowering your shoulders and twisting and pulling back your shoulder blades.The neck and head may be turned with the aid of the traps. You can often feel stress in your upper traps if you work at a desk all day.

Typically, the rhomboids squeeze your shoulder blades together.Your posture will be significantly helped by strengthening your rhomboids. It's crucial to train your rhomboids to balance out all of the pushing motions you undertake throughout the day since they do the opposing action of your chest (pulling).

The muscles that support and move your scapula are another crucial set of muscles in your upper back (shoulder blade). Your rotator cuff muscles are the collective name given to all of these muscles. They enable motions including elevation, depression, retraction, protraction, upward rotation, and downward rotation, in addition to aiding in shoulder stabilization. Fundamentally, your shoulder blades and rotator cuff muscles are in charge of all the entertaining motions you may do with your shoulders.

Prior to Lifting:

When doing the moves in this chapter, keep your core tight. To ensure proper form, you may also practice each of these moves in front of a mirror or on videotape.

WARM-UP
T-SPINE ROTATION

Warming up and stretching your upper back is crucial for improving the mobility of your thoracic spine, also known as the T-spine, which is located in the center of your back. If you sit for a long time or have other muscle imbalances, the middle of your back may become less flexible.By doing this stretch, you may get some of your mobility back, which will help you lift weights better in the long run.

1. Lean to one side. With your hands pushed together, extend both arms straight out in front of your chest.
2. Straighten your bottom leg while bending the upper leg's knee to a 90-degree angle.
3. Twist through your midback and head so that your eyes are following your hand as you slowly take your upper hand and open it to the other side of the floor.
4. At the conclusion of the stretch, your upper knee should still be bent and your arms should be straight at 180 degrees.
5. Repeat on the other side after slowly returning to the beginning position.

EXERCISE
BENT OVER ROW

Additional Muscles Successful: Core, Biceps

This exercise helps to improve posture and especially targets the rhomboids. Also, it's an excellent workout for strengthening the deadlifting movement pattern. Due to the use of your middle and lower back muscles, a powerful bent-over row will aid in enhancing the strength of your other back workouts.

1. Holding dumbbells at your sides or a barbell in front of you with your hands clutching the bar just outside your thighs, stand tall with your feet under your hips.

2.Hinge at the hips and tuck your chin into your chest. When you do this, try to keep your back as flat and straight as you can. Your hands should be facing each other, and the weights should be parallel to your chest at this point.

3.Row the weights up until they are at your ribcage while simultaneously bending both elbows. At the peak of this motion, squeeze your shoulder blades together.

4. With your elbows straight, slowly bring the weights back to their starting position.

5.When you're done with all the reps while bending forward, get back to the starting position.

Raise safely by maintaining a flat back the whole time. When doing the action, avoid rounding the center of your spine or arching your lower back. Instead of engaging your upper traps, contract the muscles in your middle back. Draw your shoulder blades down and squeeze them together to do this. Maintain a neutral neck and as relaxed a set of shoulders as you can.

Making It Simpler If maintaining the bending posture is too difficult, you may support your weight on a chair with one hand while holding a dumbbell in the other. Utilize the chair to assist you in establishing the proper neutral spine posture for this exercise while stabilizing your core.

EXERCISE
REVERSE FLY

Additional Muscles: Core And Shoulders.

This exercise works some of the minor muscles in and around your rotator cuff muscles very well. It's a great way to improve your posture and strengthen your body as a whole.While it uses fewer muscle groups, this exercise is significantly harder than bent-over rows.

1. Hold dumbbells at your sides and stand with your feet hip-width apart.
2. Hinge at the hips and descend your chest toward the floor while maintaining a straight, flat back. Your hands should be facing each other, and the weights should be parallel to your chest at this point.
3. Extend both arms straight out to your sides to create a long line, keeping your arms straight and your elbows slightly bent. At the peak of the action, push your shoulder blades together and see yourself as a bird spreading its wings to fly.
4. Return the weights to the front of your chest, in the middle of your torso.

Raise Caution: Raise the weights slowly and steadily. Try not to utilize momentum to thrust your neck forward or raise your chest to lift the weights. Limit the length of your arms. Use a comfortable range of motion for the movement. Do not let your lower back arch.
Home Exercise Tip: You should attempt this workout using a resistance band. Just hold the band's opposing ends together (as opposed to holding the handles). As though you were attempting to tear the band in two, pull it apart.

EXERCISE
FARMER'S CARRY

Another exercise to help you posture-correct is this one. It's also a really practical workout since it mimics motions you already perform on a regular basis, like carrying shopping bags. The next time you carry purses or shopping bags, keep this practice in mind.

1. Hold dumbbells at your sides while standing with your feet hip-width apart.
2. Take a few steps in a straight line, then turn around and go backward.
3. To keep an upright posture while you walk, brace your core and press your shoulder blades together. When carrying your dumbbells, you should try to maintain the best posture you can. You should be able to feel your core contracting and shoulders slightly lowering as you walk with heavy enough weights.
Raise Caution: Before and after the workout, pay particular attention to how you take up and set down your dumbbells. While doing this, use proper squat form. While holding the weights, try to keep your back straight.

Make It Difficult: Use just one weight for the workout; this will make you engage your core and your balance more. Walking more slowly might also make it more difficult.
Home Exercise Tip: There are several objects that may be used for a farmer's carry. The name comes from the fact that farmers often use this method to move different things around their farms.Be inventive and see what you can carry about your house, such as buckets, gardening tools, bags, and luggage.

STRETCH
CAT-COW

Another effective exercise to improve thoracic mobility is the cat-cow. It is especially beneficial for those with rounded spines and/or forward-facing shoulders. You may learn how to use Cat-Cow to bring your spine back to a neutral posture for exercises like weightlifting.

1. Begin in a quadruped posture (on your hands and knees with your palms flat on the ground), with your knees precisely under your hips, your toes flat on the floor, and your wrists tucked under your shoulders.
To resemble a cat, you should droop your head, arch your back, and tuck your hips.
3. To create the shape of a cow, lift your head forward and arch your lower back by pushing your stomach toward the floor.
4. Continue the motion, smoothly transitioning from cow to cat.

LESS BACK

Back discomfort in the lower back is common. This may sometimes be brought on by weak lower back muscles or, more often, a weak core. It's crucial to strengthen your lower back by engaging in stability-building functional activities if you want to prevent lower back discomfort. The lower back should be a stable joint, according to the "joint-by-joint method" (a belief that the body is composed of alternating stable and mobile joints). In order to make up for a lack of mobility in your hip joints or thoracic spine (T-spine), your lower back will forgo stability in favor of more movement. As you can see, sometimes the problem is not a lack of power but a lack of steadiness.

If you were unsure or worried about lifting weights to help your lower back, the above reason should put your mind at ease. Everything in this chapter is designed to make your core stronger and your lower back more stable. The key to preventing general lower back discomfort is functional strength.

Prior to Lifting:

When doing the moves in this chapter, keep your core tight. To ensure proper form, you may also practice each of these moves in front of a mirror or on videotape.

WARM-UP
T-SPINE ROTATION

Since a mobile T-spine will help your lower back stabilize when you complete the exercises in this chapter, it is included again as a warm-up for your lower back. Keep in mind that your body functions as one continuous kinetic chain. Each muscle and joint contributes to the movement that is sought.

1. Lean to one side. With your hands pushed together, extend both arms straight out in front of your chest.

2. Straighten your bottom leg while bending the upper leg's knee to a 90-degree angle.

3. Twist through your midback and head so that your eyes are following your hand as you slowly take your upper hand and open it to the other side of the floor.

4. At the conclusion of the stretch, your upper knee should still be bent and your arms should be straight at 180 degrees.

5. Repeat on the other side after slowly returning to the beginning position.

EXERCISE
DUMBBELL BIRD-DOG

Additional Muscles Worked: Shoulders, Glutes, and Core
A well-executed Bird-Dog is a powerful core stabilizer. It teaches your lower back how to maintain stability while your arms and legs are in motion. To successfully complete the majority of weightlifting workouts, you must possess this ability.

1. Begin by getting down on your hands and knees and holding a dumbbell out in front of you. Put your shoulders over your wrists and your hips above your knees.

2. To keep your back stable in a neutral position, keep your midback from rounding and your lower back from arching.Moreover, your neck should be straight, not bent or extended. Imagine a pole that you want to keep in touch with with your head, midback, and tailbone while it is on your back.

3. With your palm facing inward, stretch your arm straight forward while holding the dumbbell in front of you. Extend the opposing leg behind you at the same moment. Maintain your flexed feet and

simulate kicking the wall behind you with your lifted heel.

4.Continue to maintain a neutral spine while you simultaneously lower your hand and your foot to the ground.

5. Continue on the other side.

Lifting safely means putting your spine in a neutral position and keeping it there the whole time. Your spine should naturally curve into a neutral position, which is called a neutral spine. There shouldn't be any very extreme flexion or extension.

Making It Simpler Use less weight or restrict your range of motion while doing this activity.

Make It Harder: Do pull-ups to work your whole back and develop strength. By mounting a pull-up bar to your doorframe, you may do them in your own house. A chin-up max that you can buy and install on your pull-up bar will allow you to do aided pull-ups at home. If you are unable to do pull-ups, most gyms also provide an assisted pull-up machine.

EXERCISE
GOOD MORNING

The erector muscles in the lower back are strengthened by doing this exercise. If you've mastered the Deadlift hip-hinge pattern and don't have a lower back ailment right now, you should try it.

1. Achieve a hip-width distance between your feet while standing upright.

2. Close to your body, hold a dumbbell with two hands at your chest.

3. As you bend and drop your chest toward the floor, maintain your back flat and hinge at your hips. After your hamstrings have had a decent stretch, stop.

4. Squeeze your glutes to stand up straight.

Raise Caution: While you make this motion, keep your back flat. Avoid bending or arching your back. Only descend as far as your hip mobility will allow. Stop and turn back upright if you see your lower back rounding at all.

Making It Simpler Do this motion without any weight.
You may make it harder by adding additional weight to yourself by supporting a barbell on your upper back. The workout is also more challenging when you carry the weight on your back rather than your front.

STRETCH
CHILD'S POSE

The shoulders, upper and lower back, and hips may all be stretched with this exercise. Most people also find it relaxing, and it may help increase the range of motion in the hips and ankles.All of these joints' increased mobility might make your lower back feel less strained.

1. On the floor, crouch down with your hands under your shoulders and your knees under your hips, or broader if more comfortable.
2. Spread your toes out flat on the ground, facing down. When you swing your hips back toward your heels, extend both of your arms forward.
3. As you raise your arms forward and your hips back, try to straighten your back as much as you can. As you reach the stretch's maximum range, your forehead should be down and your chest should be parallel to the floor.
4.After you've had enough stretching, push your hips and shoulders forward to get back into the quadruped posture.

OBLIQUES AND ABDOMINALS

Everyone strives to retain their abs after gaining them because they want them to seem flat. The rectus abdominis, generally known as the "six-pack," is the muscle group that most people picture when you hear "abs." Your genes decide how the rectus abdominis fascia looks and where it is on your body.Because of this, some individuals have lengthy abs while others have square abs. Also, this explains why some individuals naturally have a six-pack while others have an eight- or four-pack. Everyone has abs, but for the most part, people can't see them because of a layer of fat covering them. No matter how hard you train your abs, neither their number nor form will alter. You must improve your diet and lose body fat if you want to be able to see your rectus abdominis.

There are four groups of muscles in your abdomen. These are the external obliques, rectus abdominis, internal obliques, and transverse abdominis, moving inward from the outer layer. The deepest abdominal muscle, the transverse abdominis, surrounds the core from front to back and runs between the ribs and the hips. Your most crucial abdominal muscle is this one! It is responsible for stabilizing your lower back and pelvic floor, as well as your lower back and organs. It also helps with forceful exhalation. Your lower back is stabilized by this muscle, which cooperates with your pelvic floor muscles and other abdominal muscles. Your ability to lift heavier weights and your core stability will both be significantly improved by strengthening this muscle.

You may bend and twist from side to side with the help of your external and internal obliques, which are situated on the sides of your trunk. If you engage in daily tasks that call for rotation, it's crucial to build these muscle groups.

Prior to Lifting:

To target deep core muscles, keep in mind to engage your core by pulling your belly button toward your spine. Act as if you're attempting to inflate a balloon or fog up a window as you exhale. You should always feel your core engaged while doing these exercises, so keep that in mind. If you start to feel pain in your hip flexors or lower back, stop the exercise, reset, and focus on getting your core to work.

WARM-UP
PLANK

This exercise is fantastic for engaging your transverse abdominis and other deep core muscles. Your core will get considerably stronger as a result, and it will be better equipped to support you while you complete other workouts. As your core should be engaged throughout all lifts, planking is often a terrific warm-up exercise to do before exercising any muscle group.

1.Start prone (on your stomach), with your knees and toes on the ground and your elbows exactly beneath your shoulders. Around hip distance should separate your feet.
2. Maintaining a level hip and shoulder posture, slowly raise your knees off the floor.
3. Imagine trying to keep your head, midback, and butt in touch while carrying a pole on your back.Your lower back shouldn't be arched at all.
4. Strongly contract your glutes and firmly push your forearms into the ground. 5. Release your knees to the ground after you've finished the exercise, or you may pretend to pull your elbows to your rib cage by not moving them.

EXERCISE
SIDE BRIDGE:

Glutes, Shoulders, and Other Additional Muscles Worked

Your deep core muscles, including your obliques, will benefit from this workout. Moreover, the movement pattern supports the hip extension required for deadlifts and squats. The hip extension observed in power exercises is simulated by raising your hips off the ground while placing your front foot forward.

1. Place your top foot in front of your bottom foot while lying on your side with your legs straight. Make sure your elbow is just below your shoulder and that you are lying on your forearm.
2. Drive your upper hip up toward the ceiling while slowly raising your hips off the floor.
3. You have the option of keeping your opposite hand at your side or lifting it such that it is parallel to your shoulder in the air.
Making It Simpler Your lower leg may remain on the ground. Bring your bottom foot behind you by extending your top leg and bending your bottom knee.
If you want to make it tougher, you may pull up your top leg and hover while in the complete Side Bridge, or you can make it harder by bending that knee inward toward your chest. Put your foot back where it was at the beginning, on the ground. Repeat as many times or for as many seconds as you want. To make this a weighted exercise, you may additionally hold a dumbbell in your upper hand.

EXERCISE
HOLLOW-BODY HOLDS

This is a fantastic maneuver to practice synchronizing your upper and lower halves. If practicing handstands is one of your goals, it's a great method to get your body ready for them.

1. Sit flat on your back with your legs straight and your arms outstretched over your head. Keep your hands facing each other and your feet together.

2. Lift your feet off the ground a few inches and slowly lift your shoulder blades off the floor, stretching your hands up and out behind you.

3. Continue to hold yourself in this raised posture while trying to keep your lower back from arching. Maintain your lower back firmly planted on the ground.

4. Go back to the beginning.

Raise Caution: You should be aware of how you are utilizing your body weight even if you are not lifting any weights throughout this workout. Be cautious to maintain a relaxed neck and shoulders. Keep your head and neck from moving forward as you lift your shoulder blades off the floor. Ensure there is no gap between your back and the ground when you raise your feet off the floor to further safeguard your lower back. Remember to breathe normally during your hold.

Making It Simpler To alter the grip, maintain your hands at your sides rather than raising them over your head. Reach your arms toward your heels as you elevate your body into the hold position, and try to make your body as long as you can.

Make It Difficult: With both hands, grasp a dumbbell.

EXERCISE
LOWER-LEG LIFT

You can train your abs with this difficult workout without bending your spine. To prevent straining your back, you must absolutely avoid flexing your spine.

1. Lay on your back with your hands at your sides and your legs at a comfortable height. Ensure that the bottom of your back is flat on the floor.

2. Slowly squat down until you feel your lower back begin to arch, then stop. Your goal should be to gain enough strength to lift your feet a few inches off the ground.

3. Pull your legs back up to the beginning position while contracting your abdominals.

Raise Caution: During the whole movement, maintain a flat lower back on the ground. Your lower back shouldn't at any point be arched. Keep your neck and shoulders as loose as you can while keeping your head down to the ground. You should stop this exercise and focus on strengthening your core with the other exercises recommended in this chapter if you are unable to complete it without arching your back.

Making It Simpler Just below your butt, where your lower back and tailbone meet, place your hands. While you make the motion, keep your hands in that location. You'll be able to complete your leg lifts without using your hands as your core control improves.

To make it harder, rise and drop your legs while holding a barbell or dumbbell over your chest.

EXERCISE
DEAD BUG

For people of all fitness levels, the Dead Bug exercise is great for the abs. Most persons with back pain may do this action safely, and it will assist in strengthening the core, which may help to lessen back discomfort.

1. Lay flat on your back. Your feet and calves should be parallel to the ground as you lift your knees over your hips.

2. Raise your arms straight up in the air over your chest.

3. As you stretch your left arm back behind your head and your right leg straight out in front of you, keep your lower back fully flat on the ground.

4. Repeat on the other side after returning your hand and foot to the

beginning position. You should resemble a dying insect with this back-and-forth movement of your limbs and legs.

5. As you carry out the motion, keep your head down to the floor.

Make It Difficult: Lay a foam roller over the tops of your thighs while holding it in place with your hands, if you have one. Firmly rub the foam roller over your thighs. Now remove one hand from the foam roller and raise it over your head while extending the other leg. Your other arm and leg should still be firmly in touch with the foam roller while you move the affected arm and leg. On the other side, repeat For this phase, you may either use a stability ball or add weight by holding dumbbells in each hand.

Home Exercise Tip: Here's a tip on how to tilt your pelvis when doing ab workouts like this one so that your lower back stays parallel to the ground: Place a towel that has been lengthwise rolled beneath your lower back. Its ends should protrude over your sides and be positioned in the small of your back, between your buttocks and rib cage. Raise your legs and use your lower back to try to crush the towel. Now, while keeping your legs up, grasp the towel and try to move it out from behind you. Practice until you are unable to yank the towel from behind you any longer.

EXERCISE
RUSSIAN TWIST

WORKING ARMS AND QUAD MUSCLES

Your obliques and lower abs will be well-targeted by this technique. Also, it's a useful exercise for teaching your body to rotate from the T-spine rather than your lower back, which is safer for your lower back.

1. Kneel down on the floor with your feet together. Using both hands, hold a dumbbell at your chest.

2. Lift your feet off the ground while you lean back slightly.

3. Rotate the weight to the right side of your body by twisting using

your T-spine and obliques rather than simply your arms. Return to your center and turn to the left. Do a head turn so that you can follow the weight with your eyes.

4. Keep swiveling from side to side. While you do this, try to prevent your legs from swaying.

For safe lifting, you should always keep your back straight and let your neck and shoulders relax.Twist from your midback, not from your lower back.

Making It Simpler Keep your feet firmly planted. You may also simplify it by not utilizing a weight and concentrating just on perfecting the side-to-side motion.

STRETCH

COBRA

Your abdominal muscles may cramp up just like other muscles. To prevent this, you should spread them out in between sets. Cobra is a terrific exercise for this since it extends the front of the body.

1. When lying on your stomach, place your hands close to your chest with your arms bent. Keep your feet close together and plant your feet firmly on the ground.

2. Put your hands on the ground and lift your chest off the floor while extending your elbows. While you do this, the ground should still be under your hips.

3. When you feel a decent stretch in your abdominals and no pain in your lower back, stop extending your back. Return to the floor and let go.

BICEPS AND TRICEPS

The biceps and triceps are the muscles that come to mind when discussing weight training, despite the fact that your arms are made up of several other muscles. Some women fear becoming "bulky" because they fear lifting weights and believe they have weak arms.Women cannot acquire bulk without following a very precise regimen of arm exercises and a very specialized diet that is high in calories. This is true of a woman's physique in general, but especially of her arms. You may develop greater strength and tone your arms by lifting weights. Do you like to be able to carry something comfortably and easily, or do you prefer to be able to assertively flex your arms while giving someone three seconds to back away from you? This chapter is for you if you can affirmatively say yes to any of these questions.

The muscles in your arms that face forward while your arms are relaxed at your sides are known as biceps. While your arms are relaxed, the muscle group on the rear of your arms is known as the triceps. You have three triceps heads in addition to two biceps heads. One group is called "bi-" and the other "tri-" because of this. The long head and the short head are the two heads of the biceps (biceps brachii). To aid in somewhat distinct motions, the long head and short head emerge from two separate scapular sites. The long head, lateral head, and medial head are the three heads of the triceps (triceps brachii). The long head comes from the scapula, whereas the lateral and medial heads come from various locations on the humerus (arm bone). This indicates that each tricep head slightly alters how the arm is moved. The triceps and biceps function in opposition to one another. Your elbow is flexed by your biceps and extended by your triceps. This implies that whether you do a push or pull exercise like push-ups, chest presses, pull-ups, or rows, your biceps and triceps are engaged. While you'll burn more calories by utilizing bigger muscle groups, using your arms as part of a larger muscle group is more efficient. Nonetheless, it is advised that you do a few solitary arm workouts if you are especially trying to add more definition to your arms.

Before You Lift: While doing the exercises in this chapter, keep your core tight. To ensure proper form, you may also practice each of these moves in front of a mirror or on videotape.

PLANK

WARM-UP

UP-DOWN

This exercise is a terrific way to get your heart rate up and your arms' circulation flowing. Your arms will benefit from the up-and-down motion as you get ready for your weightlifting sessions.
1. Get into a low plank position on the floor with your toes hip-width apart and your elbows right under your shoulders.
2. While keeping your left forearm on the ground, walk up onto your right hand. You need to be doing a half-pushup.
3. Climb up onto your left hand so that your hands are now on the ground under your shoulders and you are in the top push-up position.
4. Drop one arm back to the floor to get back on one forearm.
5. Drop the opposite arm until both forearms are flat on the floor, returning you to the low plank position.

Traditional Bicep Curl Exercise Additional Muscles That Worked:

Forearms
This type of curl is great for making your muscles stronger and more defined, especially in the biceps of each arm.It's also excellent for

building up your biceps' strength so you can lift larger objects while doing back workouts.

1. Hold a barbell in front of you at your thighs with your hands up while standing with your feet hip-width apart. Dumbbells are another option for this exercise. Dumbbells held at your sides.
2. Raise the weight toward your chest while slowly bending your elbows. Just before your chest, stop.
3. Let the weight fall back down to touch your thighs by extending at the elbows.

Raise Caution: While you carry out this exercise, relax your neck and shoulders. During the exercise, maintain your elbows at your sides. They shouldn't go ahead or behind. In order to prevent circulation problems, it's also critical that you stand with your knees slightly bent but not locked.

Make It Difficult: Take 1 second to raise the weight, then 3 seconds to lower it. Since you put more muscle into the downward motion as you dropped the weight, you should take longer. As an alternative, isolate each arm using dumbbells. Dumbbell curls that are performed with the dumbbells externally rotated will more effectively target the short (inner) and long (outer) heads of the bicep muscles and activate more muscle fibers, which results in the development of more muscle.

Hammer Curl Exercise: Additional Muscles Worked: Forearms

Hammer curls work a different area of your biceps than traditional bicep curls do.They focus on the brachialis, a muscle in the arm that is different from the biceps and is in charge of external rotation. They also work on the brachioradialis and the long heads of the biceps. Hammer curls will strengthen your wrists while also assisting with the growth of your biceps.

1. Hold a dumbbell in each hand with the palms facing inward while standing with your feet hip-width apart.

2. Bend your elbows and lift the two weights to your chest. Keep your hands pointing toward one another, inward. (You would lift your glass in the same way to take a sip.)

3. Return the weights to your sides.

Lifting Safely: It's important to stand with your knees slightly bent but not locked if you don't want circulation problems.

Raise one arm at a time to make it simpler. It will be simpler to do this than to attempt to raise both at once.

Make It Difficult: Lift the weights for one second, then lower them for three seconds.

More muscles were activated as a result of exercise trigger point kickback.

Forearms

The backs of the arms are effectively worked out with this great workout. When you use dumbbells to isolate the effort in each arm, neither side is compensating for the other, and you can discover that one arm has stronger triceps muscles.

1. Take a hip-width stance while keeping your knees slightly bent. Your hands should be pointing inward toward your thighs while you hold the dumbbells at your sides.

2. Hinge from your hips and gently lower your chest. Maintain this posture while keeping your spine long by gazing down at the ground a few feet in front of you.

3. To position the weights near your upper ribs, bend your elbows while simultaneously bringing them up behind you.

4. To raise the dumbbells to your shoulders, extend your elbows straight back without elevating your chest or rotating your shoulders.

5. To return the weights to their initial position, bend your elbows.

Making It Simpler Instead of attempting to lift both weights at once, lift one at a time.

To make it harder, hold your stance after completely extending your elbows for one second before letting go. To make the movement more difficult, you may also slow it down.

EXERCISE

TRICEP OVERHEAD EXTENSION IS AN

In this workout, you target your triceps muscles differently by extending your arms upward while keeping your shoulders still. This activity will also increase your shoulder mobility. Nevertheless, use one of the other triceps workouts listed if you have a shoulder ailment or restricted mobility.

1. Stand with your feet separated by your shoulders.
2. Make a diamond-shaped pattern between the palms of your hands and extend your arms upwards while holding one weight in each hand.
3. Bend your elbows so that your head is squarely behind the weight.
4. To return the weight above, straighten your elbows.
Raise Caution: When executing this exercise, keep your rib cage down and avoid arching your back. (Consider avoiding exaggerating your chest.)
Make It Difficult: At the peak of the exercise, hold for an additional two seconds before bringing the weight back down behind your head.

EXERCISE

OVERHEAD

Other muscles worked include the core and shoulders. While working your triceps, this exercise is a great way to increase your core stability and shoulder mobility. With only one motion, you get three fantastic advantages!

1. With your knees bent and your feet flat on the ground, lie on your back on the ground.
2. Hold one weight over your chest, forming a diamond shape between your palms, and stretching your elbows.
3. Slightly bend your elbows, then raise the weight as high as you can without letting your lower back arch or your ribcage rise.
4. Push the weight forward, crossing it across your chest, to put your shoulders back in their initial position.
Raise: To do this exercise safely, don't let your lower back arch and don't let your shoulders go too far back.Work just within a range of motion that is comfortable for you until your shoulder mobility improves.
Make It Difficult: Lift your feet off the ground and cross your knees over your hips. More core stability will be necessary for this.

BICEP STRETCH WHILE STANDING

This is one way to stretch your biceps after lifting weights by yourself so they don't cramp up.If you work out your biceps, you may find that your elbows stay bent because your biceps have shrunk.To get your biceps back to their natural length, you must stretch them. Your shoulders may round forward as a result of tight, shortened biceps, which will also limit the range of motion in your shoulders.

1. Place your feet hip-width apart and stand.
2. Place your hands behind your back, entwine them, and turn your elbows inward so that your palms are facing the ground.
3. Raise your arms behind you while extending your shoulders until you feel a stretch in your biceps.
4. Go back to the beginning position with your hands.

STRETCH

TRICEP STRETCH OVERHEAD

To prevent arm cramps at the back of your arms, do this stretch right away after working out your triceps. You should do this stretch to avoid tennis elbow, which is pain in the elbow joint caused by overusing your forearms or doing the same motions over and over with your elbow bent.

1. Place your feet hip-width apart and stand.
2. Raise one arm above you, bending the elbow so that the hand is near the shoulder.
3. To experience a wonderful triceps stretch, raise the opposite arm and push down and back on the elbow of the bent arm.
4. Release, then do the same on the other side.

SHOULDERS

The muscles in the shoulders are strong but very delicate. The rotator cuff muscles, trapezius, rhomboids, serratus anterior, levator scapulae, and pectoralis minor are some of the muscles of the shoulder girdle. Contrary to popular belief, the shoulder is made up of more muscles than just the deltoids. Many additional muscles, such as the latissimus dorsi, sometimes known as the "lats," also influence the shoulder joint. Your shoulder may be moved in one of the following ways using each of these muscles: flexion, extension, internal rotation, external rotation, adduction, and abduction. As you can see, the shoulder is a complicated region that calls for a lot of body synergy.

Your shoulder's ball-and-socket joint is shallow, so it doesn't have as much bony support as your hip joint does (the other ball-and-socket joint in your body). As a result, the shoulder needs greater muscle support to remain stable. Without sufficient muscle protection, the shoulder is vulnerable to harm, including dislocations. Additionally, due to extended sitting, the majority of individuals have internally rotated shoulders. The shoulder joint is more vulnerable to injury as a result of this limitation on the shoulder's normal range of motion. So, it's crucial to improve both your shoulder mobility and the stability of the muscles that support your shoulder joint. Stability comes after mobility. In order to ensure that you have complete shoulder range of motion before starting your weightlifting regimen, focus on warming up your shoulders with the warm-up exercises in this chapter.

Before You Lift: While doing the exercises in this chapter, keep your core tight. To ensure proper form, you may also practice each of these moves in front of a mirror or on videotape.

CROSS-BODY ARM SWING

Your shoulder joint's blood flow will be aided by this motion. To prevent damage, you should lubricate your joints well before engaging in any shoulder workouts.

1. Attain a T-position while standing with your feet hip-width apart and your arms at your sides.
2. Swing your arms forward until they form a cross in the middle of your body.
3. Return your arms to their open, extended state. Swing your arms back out to your sides at chest height and forward again.

WALL ANGEL

To improve the range of motion in your shoulders, try this stretch. Also, it aids in preventing internal shoulder rotation, commonly known as shoulder rounding, which is a common side effect of spending the most of the day sitting down.

1. Place your rib cage down and butt against the wall as you lean against the wall.
2. To make a goal post with your arms, bring them up against the wall, elbows bent at a 90-degree angle and at shoulder height.
3. Raise your arms slowly until your elbows are straight and your hands are over your head while attempting to keep touch with the wall.
4. Drop your hands back down to the ground, bringing your elbows back to a 90-degree angle.

EXERCISE

SHOULDER PRESSES

One of the basic movement patterns that people learn from birth is this one. While it's one of the most popular vertical press exercises, you shouldn't execute it if your shoulders are injured or have restricted range of motion.

1. Hold a barbell or dumbbells in both palms while standing with your feet shoulder-width apart.
2. To create a 90-degree angle with your elbows, raise your elbows to shoulder height and position your wrists over them.
3. Raise the weights over your head while extending your elbows completely.
4. Go back to the beginning posture with your arms.
Raise Caution: When you pump the weights into the air, avoid arching your lower back. While you push the weights above, keep your neck in a neutral position and your ribs down.
Making It Simpler Less core activation is needed if you raise one weight at a time.
Home Exercise Tip: Use a resistance band for this workout. Just put your feet on the band and raise your arms over your head. More resistance will be produced if you stand on the band with two feet as opposed to just one.

EXERCISE

IRON CROSS

This exercise can work the three heads of your deltoid muscle, which is located at the top of your shoulder.

1. Hold the dumbbells in front of you with your hands facing down while you stand with your feet shoulder-width apart.
2. Extend your arms straight in front of you to shoulder height with the dumbbells.
3. While maintaining the dumbbells at shoulder height, make a T with your arms by extending them laterally (out to the sides).
4. Straighten your arms out again and place them by your sides.
5. To create the T, raise your arms straight up laterally, pausing when your hands are at shoulder height.
6. While maintaining your arms straight and the dumbbells at shoulder height, move your arms towards the middle of your body.
7. To return the dumbbells to the beginning position, lower both arms back down along the front of your chest.
Live securely: While you carry out this action, avoid bending your lower back. At no time throughout this exercise should you lift your hands higher than your shoulders.
Resistance bands may be used to execute this exercise at home.
Making It Simpler Do lateral rises and/or front raises instead of the complete Iron Cross. The initial phase of the action consists of front lifts. (Lift the weights to your shoulders, then drop them to your waist.) The second part of the action consists of lateral rises.

BICEPS WERE

The little shoulder muscles that were not targeted in the previous two exercises are the focus of this exercise. It is a frontal plane movement that puts more of an emphasis on your shoulders' front and midsection. In order to help define the shoulders further, bodybuilders often do this action. If your shoulders are unhealthy or your posture is poor, it is not advised. If you have any contraindications, think about doing a more practical workout, like the ones already mentioned.

1. Stand with your feet shoulder-width apart and dumbbells or a barbell in front of you at your thighs, holding them with your hands shoulder-width apart and palms facing inward.
2. Bend your elbows and lift the weights to chest height. Consider using your elbows to attempt to form the shape of a clothes hanger.
3.Return to the beginning position with your arms extended, maintaining the weights close to your body the whole time.
Raise Caution: While you carry out this exercise, avoid bending your lower back. If you experience any prickling or pain in the front of your shoulder, stop. When you bring the weights to chest height, imagine pressing your shoulder blades together on your back, akin to a broad row. By doing this, you'll be able to lessen some of the stress that the shoulders' internal rotation causes.
Making It Simpler Raise one dumbbell at a time as opposed to all at once.
Home Exercise Tip: You may perform this workout using a resistance band.

STRETCHING

In order to restore the muscles to their previous length, it is as vital to stretch the shoulder joint after exercise as it is to warm it up. You may preserve the correct joint range of motion by doing this.

1. Place your arms at your sides and stand.
2. Lift one arm over your head, maintaining it straight, and cross it over to the other side of your body.
3. Grasp the arm that crosses your body just past the elbow with the opposing hand.
4. Pull the arm in such that your shoulder and triceps are stretched while you do so.
5. Let go, then repeat on the other side.

EXERCISE PROGRAMS

I put everything together here so you may construct and have good workouts. While exercising, it's crucial to have a plan in place so that you can monitor your development as a weightlifter. Also, it prevents you from worrying about what to do next throughout your workout and keeps you focused on the exercise routines. The information on reps, sets, and exercise tempo that you will find on the following pages will help you create your own workouts. You will also find examples of weekly programming and various sample workouts for your entire body, upper body, and lower body that you can use as a starting point or as inspiration for creating your own workout program.

Programming

The process of programming is highly complicated. To help you design a fitness plan that is effective for you, I highly advise that you seek the advice of a licensed personal trainer. This is crucial since there are many different methods to program and it might be tough for a newbie to figure out which sorts of programs will work best for you and your objectives. After being assessed by a fitness expert, you'll have a stronger foundation from which to learn how to design and implement your own programs.

I assumed that circuit training and supersets were the best ways to build strength and lose fat when making example programs for this book.I suggest putting upper body exercises into four groups: vertical pushes, vertical pulls, horizontal pushes, and horizontal pulls.You can make sure you train every muscle group by doing this. It may be difficult to fit certain muscle groups into this rigid mold, but as you start to discover which muscles are typically engaged during each movement pattern, the classifications will start to make more sense. A vertical push would be, for instance, a shoulder press.

An upright row, which is a vertical draw, is still a shoulder workout. Here is where the rule becomes a little bit complex.

It is advised that you divide your lower-body workouts into knee-dominant and hip-dominant motions. Exercises that focus on your knee often include knee flexion and extension. Exercises that emphasize the hips are those that often include hip flexion and extension, such as hip hinge motions. For individuals who can only train a few days each week, I've also included total-body exercises. tempo, repetitions, and sets

To get stronger, it is recommended that you do 3 to 5 sets of 5 to 8 reps for each exercise.For each exercise, the pace should be around 3 seconds up and 3 seconds down. After every set, be careful to relax for 90 to 2 minutes.

Progression
You'll want to vary your exercises a little bit each week as you become better at them. For instance, if you began with 3 sets of 5 reps in week 1, you may go up to 3 sets of 8 in week 2. You might also continue with 3 sets of 5, but use heavier weights. To make sure that your strength training program is progressing and you are not plateauing, you should alter the sets, reps, pace, or length of rest each week. It is also vital that you modify one item at a time. Your body will get confused if you attempt to adjust too many things at once, which will hinder its capacity to adapt and become stronger.

Equipment
If you're looking to gain strength, you'll need a set of medium and a set of heavy dumbbells, as well as a barbell that you can add or subtract weight from, for each exercise and the following training routines in this book. to start a. The a b.............. You should feel as if you could only do one or two more repetitions with heavy weights. Using free weights, you may gradually raise your load to train your

muscles harder, yet many of these exercises can be performed with body weight to regress (or make them easier).

Days of Rest and Rehabilitation

For optimal rest and muscle healing, it's advised to take a day or two off between each exercise. You may start working out on consecutive days after you are acclimated to weightlifting and have a better understanding of programming. You should still take at least one recovery day each week, and if you can, try to take two days off for each muscle group.

Cooldowns and Warm-Ups

As stated at the start of this book, warm-ups and cool-downs shouldn't be neglected. Your body needs to be warmed up and cooled down in order to recuperate and avoid injuries. Warm-up and cool-down exercises are included in the plans that are offered later in the book.

Scheduling

I've included a few ideas of how your exercise week may look depending on your training availability on the following pages. You'll see that on days when I don't lift weights, I've added rest days and cardio choices. These examples might serve as a guide on how to organize your weeks in a manner that fits your schedule the best. I advise planning out your exercises for the next week by sitting down one evening every week—possibly Sunday before a new week starts. This will guarantee that you set aside a particular time for training and keep you accountable to yourself and your training so that nothing unforeseen arises and prevents you from exercising.

Here's a 10 week workout plan that you can try:

Weeks 1-2: Build a Strong Foundation
Day 1: Full-body workout (squats, lunges, push-ups, pull-ups, planks)
Day 2: Rest or light cardio (30 minutes of walking or cycling)
Day 3: Full-body workout (deadlifts, bench press, rows, chin-ups, bridges)
Day 4: Rest or light cardio
Day 5: Full-body workout (step-ups, dips, lat pulldowns, hamstring curls, Russian twists)
Day 6: Rest or light cardio
Day 7: Rest

Weeks 3-4: Increase Intensity
Day 1: Upper body workout (bench press, military press, pull-ups, dips, bicep curls)
Day 2: Rest or light cardio
Day 3: Lower body workout (squats, deadlifts, lunges, calf raises, bridges)
Day 4: Rest or light cardio
Day 5: Upper body workout (dumbbell press, rows, chin-ups, tricep extensions, hammer curls)
Day 6: Rest or light cardio
Day 7: Rest

Weeks 5-6: High-Intensity Interval Training (HIIT)
Day 1: HIIT cardio (30 seconds all-out effort, 30 seconds rest, repeat for 20 minutes)
Day 2: Rest or light cardio
Day 3: HIIT strength training (burpees, push-ups, squats, jumping lunges, mountain climbers)
Day 4: Rest or light cardio
Day 5: HIIT cardio (sprints, cycling, rowing, or jumping rope)

Day 6: Rest or light cardio
Day 7: Rest

Weeks 7-8: Plyometrics and Explosive Training
Day 1: Plyometric circuit (box jumps, jump squats, jump lunges, burpees, tuck jumps)
Day 2: Rest or light cardio
Day 3: Explosive strength training (power cleans, snatches, kettlebell swings, box jumps, broad jumps)
Day 4: Rest or light cardio
Day 5: Plyometric circuit
Day 6: Rest or light cardio
Day 7: Rest

Weeks 9-10: Endurance and Conditioning
Day 1: Endurance workout (jogging, cycling, swimming, rowing, or elliptical for 30-60 minutes)
Day 2: Rest or light cardio
Day 3: Conditioning workout (sled pushes, tire flips, battle ropes, farmer's walk, agility ladder)
Day 4: Rest or light cardio
Day 5: Endurance workout
Day 6: Rest or light cardio
Day 7: Rest

Repeat this cycle for the remaining weeks, adjusting the exercises and weight as necessary. Remember to always warm up before each workout and stretch afterward to prevent injury. And make sure to listen to your body and adjust the intensity as needed.

Tips for Proper Weight Training Form

Proper posture and alignment

Proper posture and alignment are crucial for weight training, especially for women over 40. Here are some tips for maintaining proper posture and alignment during weight training:

1. Keep your head in line with your spine: Your head should be aligned with your spine, neither leaning forward nor backward. This will help prevent neck strain and injury.
2. Engage your core: Before beginning any exercise, engage your core by drawing your belly button toward your spine. This will help stabilize your spine and prevent injury.
3. Keep your shoulders back and down: Avoid hunching your shoulders forward. Instead, keep them back and down, which will help prevent upper back and neck pain.
4. Maintain a neutral spine: Avoid rounding or arching your back during exercises, as this can cause injury. Instead, maintain a neutral spine, with a slight natural curve in your lower back.
5. Keep your feet hip-width apart: When standing, keep your feet hip-width apart with your toes pointing forward. This will help maintain balance and stability.
6. Bend your knees: When lifting weights, bend your knees slightly to protect your lower back and maintain stability.
7. Use proper form: When performing exercises, use proper form and technique to avoid injury and maximize results. If you're not sure how to perform an exercise correctly, consider working with a certified personal trainer.

Remember to start with lighter weights and gradually increase the weight as you become more comfortable and proficient with the exercises. And always listen to your body – if something doesn't feel right, stop and adjust your form or weight as needed.

Breathing techniques

Breathing techniques are an important part of weight training, especially for women over 40 who may have decreased lung capacity and endurance. Proper breathing during weightlifting can help increase oxygen intake and improve performance, while also reducing the risk of injury. Here are a few breathing techniques for weight training for women over 40:

1. Inhale before the lift: Take a deep breath in before lifting the weight. This helps to stabilize the core muscles and create a solid foundation for the lift.
2. Exhale during the exertion: Exhale as you lift or push the weight, and inhale as you lower or release it. This helps to regulate your breathing and maintain proper form.
3. Use the valsalva maneuver: The valsalva maneuver involves holding your breath briefly during the lift to increase intra-abdominal pressure and support the spine. This can be helpful for heavier lifts, but should be used with caution and only with proper instruction.
4. Breathe consistently: Keep your breathing consistent throughout the set, and avoid holding your breath or taking shallow breaths. This can cause dizziness or lightheadedness, and can compromise your form and safety.

Remember to also take breaks and allow your body to recover between sets, and to consult with a certified personal trainer or healthcare professional before starting any new exercise program.

Common weight training mistakes to avoid

Weight training is an effective way for women over 40 to improve their strength, bone density, and overall health. However, there are some common mistakes that women in this age group can make while weight training. Here are some mistakes to avoid:

1. Lifting too much weight: Women over 40 may have a higher risk of injury and joint pain, so it's important to start with lighter weights and gradually increase the weight as strength improves.
2. Not using proper form: Using proper form is essential for avoiding injury and getting the most out of your workout. Make sure you learn the correct form for each exercise before you start lifting.
3. Not allowing enough recovery time: Recovery time is essential for building muscle and avoiding injury. Make sure you rest for at least 48 hours between workouts for the same muscle group.
4. Focusing only on cardio: While cardio is important for overall health, weight training is essential for building muscle and improving bone density. Make sure you incorporate both types of exercise into your routine.
5. Not varying your routine: Doing the same exercises over and over can lead to plateaus in your progress. Make sure you mix up your routine by trying new exercises or increasing the weight or reps.
6. Neglecting warm-up and cool-down: A proper warm-up and cool-down routine can help prevent injury and improve flexibility. Make sure you spend at least 5-10 minutes warming up before your workout and stretching after your workout.
7. Not fueling your body properly: Proper nutrition is essential for building muscle and recovering from workouts. Make sure you eat a balanced diet that includes plenty of protein, carbohydrates, and healthy fats.

By avoiding these common mistakes, women over 40 can enjoy the benefits of weight training while minimizing the risk of injury and maximizing their progress.

Advanced Weight Training Techniques

Progressive overload

Progressive overload is a key principle in weight training that involves gradually increasing the demands placed on the body over time. This helps to stimulate muscle growth and improve overall strength and fitness. However, for advanced weight training techniques, simply adding more weight may not always be the best way to achieve progressive overload. Here are some ways to apply progressive overload to advanced weight training techniques:

1. Volume Progression: Increase the total number of sets, reps, or exercises you perform during a workout. For example, you can gradually increase the number of sets for a specific exercise or add more exercises to your workout routine.
2. Intensity Progression: Increase the difficulty or intensity of the exercise without necessarily adding more weight. This can be done by performing exercises with stricter form, slowing down the tempo of the exercise, reducing rest time between sets, or using advanced techniques such as drop sets, supersets, or rest-pause sets.
3. Range of Motion Progression: Increase the range of motion of an exercise by performing it through a greater range of motion or performing a more challenging variation of the exercise.
4. Frequency Progression: Increase the frequency with which you perform a specific exercise or workout routine. This can be done by adding an extra workout day or increasing the frequency of specific exercises within your routine.
5. Time Under Tension Progression: Increase the time that your muscles are under tension during an exercise. This can be achieved by slowing down the tempo of the exercise, using

isometric contractions, or performing exercises with lighter weights but higher reps.

By applying these different methods of progressive overload, you can continue to challenge your body and achieve new levels of strength and fitness with advanced weight training techniques.

Supersets and drop sets

Supersets and drop sets are advanced weight training techniques that can help you take your workouts to the next level. Here's a breakdown of each technique:

1. Supersets: A superset is a technique in which you perform two exercises back to back with no rest in between. For example, you could do a set of bicep curls followed immediately by a set of tricep extensions. This can increase the intensity of your workout and help you save time in the gym. There are several types of supersets, including:
   - Compound Supersets: These involve doing two exercises that work different muscle groups. For example, a bench press followed by a lat pulldown.
   - Isolation Supersets: These involve doing two exercises that work the same muscle group. For example, a bicep curl followed by a hammer curl.
   - Pre-Exhaustion Supersets: These involve doing an isolation exercise followed by a compound exercise that works the same muscle group. For example, a leg extension followed by a squat.
2. Drop sets: A drop set is a technique in which you perform a set of an exercise to failure, then immediately lower the weight and continue the set with no rest. This can help you push your muscles to fatigue and increase your overall workout volume. There are several types of drop sets, including:

- Standard Drop Sets: These involve reducing the weight by a certain percentage (usually around 20%) after each set.
- Mechanical Drop Sets: These involve changing the exercise slightly to make it easier as you fatigue. For example, you could start with a barbell curl, then switch to a hammer curl, and finish with a reverse curl.
- Rest-Pause Drop Sets: These involve taking brief rest periods (around 10-15 seconds) between each drop in weight to help you recover slightly before continuing the set.

It's important to note that both supersets and drop sets are advanced techniques that should only be used by experienced lifters. It's also important to use proper form and technique to avoid injury.

Rest-pause training

Rest-pause training is an advanced weight training technique that involves taking short rest periods during a set to allow for partial recovery, which then allows you to perform additional repetitions with the same weight. The goal of rest-pause training is to increase overall workout intensity, stimulate muscle growth, and improve strength.

To perform rest-pause training, you would first select a weight that you can lift for about 6-8 repetitions. After completing the first set, you would rest for 10-15 seconds and then attempt to perform another 2-3 repetitions with the same weight. You would continue this process of lifting, resting, and lifting again until you cannot perform any more reps.

Here are some tips for incorporating rest-pause training into your workout routine:

1. Start with a moderate weight: Rest-pause training is more intense than traditional weight training, so it's essential to start with a weight that is challenging but manageable for you.
2. Use rest-pause sparingly: Rest-pause training is a highly intense technique that can put a lot of strain on your body, so it's best to use it sparingly. One or two exercises per workout session should be enough.
3. Keep your form strict: It's important to maintain strict form when performing rest-pause sets. Avoid using momentum to help you lift the weight, as this can increase your risk of injury.
4. Monitor your rest periods: Keep track of your rest periods between sets and repetitions to ensure that you are giving your body enough time to recover.
5. Use rest-pause only for compound exercises: Rest-pause training works best for compound exercises, such as squats, bench press, and deadlifts. These exercises involve multiple muscle groups and allow you to lift heavier weights.

Overall, rest-pause training is an advanced weight training technique that can help you break through plateaus and achieve new levels of strength and muscle growth. However, it's essential to use this technique wisely and to always prioritize proper form and safety.

Tempo training

Tempo training is a technique used in advanced weight training to increase muscle strength and hypertrophy by manipulating the tempo, or speed, at which you perform each repetition of an exercise. Here are some tempo training techniques that can be used for advanced weight training:

1. Eccentric training: Eccentric training involves focusing on the lowering phase of an exercise. This can be done by slowing down the lowering phase to a count of 3-4 seconds, rather than allowing the weight to drop quickly. This technique places greater stress on the muscle fibers, leading to greater muscle damage and ultimately, increased muscle growth.
2. Pause training: Pause training involves adding a pause or hold at a specific point in the exercise. For example, during a squat, you could pause at the bottom of the squat for 2-3 seconds before rising back up. This technique increases time under tension, which can lead to greater muscle growth.
3. Tempo sets: Tempo sets involve performing a specific number of repetitions at a specific tempo. For example, you could perform 10 reps of bicep curls with a 3-second eccentric phase, a 1-second pause at the bottom, and a 1-second concentric phase. This technique can be used to target specific muscle fibers and improve mind-muscle connection.
4. Super-slow training: Super-slow training involves performing repetitions at an extremely slow pace, such as a 10-second eccentric phase, a 10-second concentric phase, and a 10-second pause. This technique can be used to increase muscle fiber recruitment and improve muscular endurance.

When incorporating tempo training into your weight training routine, it's important to start with lighter weights and gradually increase the load as you become more comfortable with the technique. Additionally, it's important to maintain proper form throughout the exercise to avoid injury.

Periodization

Periodization is a training strategy used by athletes and weightlifters to maximize their strength and muscle gains while reducing the risk of injury and burnout. Advanced weight training techniques require a well-designed periodization program to achieve the best results. Here's how to create a periodization plan for advanced weight training techniques:

1. Determine your goals: The first step is to define your long-term and short-term goals. Do you want to increase your strength, improve your muscle size, or enhance your athletic performance? Your goals will determine the focus of your periodization program.
2. Plan your training cycles: Divide your training year into cycles or phases, with each phase focusing on a specific training goal. A common periodization model is the traditional linear periodization, which divides the year into three phases: a hypertrophy phase, a strength phase, and a power phase. Another model is the undulating periodization, which alternates the training goals within each week or month.
3. Choose your advanced weight training techniques: Once you've determined your training cycles, select the advanced weight training techniques that will best help you achieve your goals. Examples of advanced weight training techniques include heavy partials, plyometrics, supersets, drop sets, and forced reps.
4. Vary your training volume and intensity: Within each training cycle, vary your training volume and intensity to prevent plateaus and overtraining. For example, during a hypertrophy phase, you may start with high volume and low intensity and gradually increase the intensity as the phase progresses.
5. Monitor your progress: Regularly assess your progress and adjust your training plan accordingly. This will help you stay motivated and make sure you're on track to reach your goals.

Remember, a well-designed periodization program can take your training to the next level and help you achieve your desired results. It's important to work with a certified personal trainer or strength and conditioning coach to design a program that meets your specific needs and goals.

Creating a Safe and Effective Weight Training Environment

Creating a safe and effective weight training environment is important to prevent injury and promote progress. Here are some key tips to consider:

1. Proper Equipment: Ensure that the weight training equipment you use is in good condition and functioning properly. Check for any signs of wear and tear, and replace any damaged equipment as soon as possible. Additionally, make sure that the equipment is appropriate for the level of weight training you are doing.
2. Proper Form: Proper form is crucial to prevent injury and promote progress. Make sure that you learn proper form for each exercise, and always use good form when lifting weights.
3. Warm-up: A good warm-up is important to prepare your body for the physical demands of weight training. Spend 5-10 minutes doing some light cardiovascular exercise, such as jogging or cycling, followed by some stretching.
4. Gradual Progression: Gradually increase the weight you lift to avoid injury and build strength over time. Don't try to lift too heavy too soon, as this can cause injury.
5. Spotting: When lifting heavy weights, it's important to have a spotter to help you if you need it. A spotter can also help you maintain proper form and prevent injury.
6. Hydration: Proper hydration is important to ensure that your body can function properly during weight training. Make sure to drink plenty of water before, during, and after your workout.
7. Rest and Recovery: Adequate rest and recovery is important to prevent injury and promote progress. Make sure to give your muscles time to recover between workouts, and get enough sleep to support muscle growth and repair.

By following these tips, you can create a safe and effective weight training environment that supports your goals and promotes progress while minimizing the risk of injury.

How to warm up and cool down

Warming up and cooling down are crucial components of any weight training routine. Here are some tips to help you create a safe and effective weight training environment:

Warming up:
- Start with 5-10 minutes of low-intensity cardiovascular exercise such as walking, jogging, or cycling to increase your heart rate and warm up your muscles.
- Follow with dynamic stretching exercises such as leg swings, arm circles, or lunges to further increase blood flow and loosen up your muscles.
- Gradually increase the intensity of your warm-up exercises, such as performing some bodyweight exercises like push-ups, squats, or lunges, to prepare your muscles for the heavier weight training to come.

Cooling down:
- After your weight training session, perform a 5-10 minute cool-down activity like light walking or cycling to gradually bring your heart rate back to a resting state.
- Follow with static stretching exercises such as holding a stretch for 15-30 seconds, focusing on the major muscle groups you worked during the weight training session, to prevent injury and increase flexibility.

- Use foam rollers, massage balls, or other self-massage tools to help relax and reduce muscle soreness after the weight training session.

Remember, warming up and cooling down is essential to help prevent injury and enhance your performance during your weight training session. Don't skip these important steps!

Importance of rest and recovery

Rest and recovery are essential components of any safe and effective weight training program. Without proper rest and recovery, the body cannot repair and rebuild the muscles that have been stressed during training. This can lead to muscle fatigue, injury, and decreased performance. Therefore, it is crucial to prioritize rest and recovery to create a safe and effective weight training environment.

Here are some specific reasons why rest and recovery are so important:

- Reducing the risk of injury: Rest and recovery allow the body to repair damaged tissues and recover from the stress of weight training. Without proper recovery, muscles may become fatigued and more prone to injury.
- Improving performance: Proper rest and recovery allow the body to regenerate energy stores and repair muscle tissue, leading to improved performance during subsequent training sessions.
- Avoiding overtraining: Overtraining can occur when the body is not given enough time to recover between workouts. This can lead to fatigue, decreased performance, and an increased risk of injury.

- Enhancing mental wellbeing: Rest and recovery can also have positive effects on mental health, reducing stress and anxiety and improving overall wellbeing.

To create a safe and effective weight training environment, it is important to prioritize rest and recovery as part of the training program. This may involve incorporating rest days into the training schedule, using proper stretching and cool-down techniques, and ensuring that participants are getting enough sleep and proper nutrition to support their recovery. By doing so, individuals can maximize the benefits of their weight training program while minimizing the risk of injury and burnout.

Injury prevention tips

Here are some injury prevention tips to help create a safe and effective weight training environment:

- Warm-up: Always start with a proper warm-up session that includes stretching and light cardiovascular exercise. This helps to prepare the muscles for the workout and reduces the risk of injury.
- Proper Technique: Ensure that you are using proper technique for each exercise. Poor technique can put unnecessary stress on your muscles and joints, which can lead to injury. Consider hiring a certified personal trainer to ensure proper technique.
- Gradual Progression: Progress your weight and volume gradually over time. Avoid making sudden jumps in weight or volume, which can increase the risk of injury.

- Appropriate Equipment: Use equipment that is appropriate for your fitness level and goals. Make sure the equipment is in good condition and is adjusted to fit your body properly.
- Spotter: Have a spotter when performing exercises that require heavy weights or involve potential risk of injury. A spotter can help you lift the weight safely and assist you in case of any mishap.
- Hydration and Rest: Stay hydrated during your workout and take enough rest between sets to allow your body to recover. Overtraining and dehydration can increase the risk of injury.
- Listen to your Body: Pay attention to your body and stop immediately if you feel any pain or discomfort. Ignoring the signs of discomfort can lead to serious injury.
- Cool-down: End your workout with a proper cool-down session that includes stretching to help your muscles relax and prevent soreness.

By following these tips, you can create a safe and effective weight training environment that will help you achieve your fitness goals while reducing the risk of injury.

Proper nutrition and hydration

Proper nutrition and hydration are essential for creating a safe and effective weight training environment. Here are some guidelines to follow:

- Hydration: Adequate hydration is crucial for safe and effective weight training. Dehydration can lead to fatigue, dizziness, and even fainting. Make sure to drink water before, during, and after your workout. The amount of water you need depends on your body weight and activity level, but as a general rule, aim for at least 8 cups (64 ounces) per day.

- Pre-Workout Nutrition: To ensure optimal performance during weight training, you need to fuel your body with the right nutrients. Eat a meal or snack that contains carbohydrates and protein about 30 minutes to an hour before your workout. Carbohydrates provide energy, while protein helps to build and repair muscle tissue. Examples of pre-workout snacks include a banana and peanut butter, Greek yogurt with fruit, or a turkey sandwich on whole-grain bread.
- Post-Workout Nutrition: After your weight training session, your body needs nutrients to repair and rebuild muscle tissue. Eating a combination of carbohydrates and protein within 30 minutes to an hour after your workout can help facilitate muscle recovery. Examples of post-workout snacks include a protein shake, a chicken and veggie stir-fry, or a tuna salad with whole-grain crackers.
- Nutrient Timing: The timing of your meals and snacks can also impact your weight training performance. Aim to eat a meal containing carbohydrates and protein about 2-3 hours before your workout. This will provide your body with the necessary energy and nutrients to power through your training session. Also, make sure to eat a snack containing carbohydrates and protein within 30 minutes to an hour after your workout to aid in muscle recovery.
- Macronutrient Balance: Your body needs a balance of carbohydrates, protein, and fat to function properly. Aim to consume a diet that is about 40% carbohydrates, 30% protein, and 30% fat. This balance will provide your body with the nutrients it needs to fuel your workouts and support muscle growth and recovery.

By following these guidelines, you can create a safe and effective weight training environment that supports optimal performance and muscle growth while minimizing the risk of injury.

Conclusion

In conclusion, weight training is a highly beneficial form of exercise for women over 40. As women age, they tend to lose muscle mass and bone density, which can lead to a host of health problems, such as osteoporosis and muscle weakness. Weight training can help to combat these issues by building and maintaining muscle mass, strengthening bones, and improving overall health and wellbeing.

In addition to the physical benefits, weight training can also have a positive impact on mental health. Studies have shown that regular exercise can help to reduce stress, improve mood, and boost self-confidence. For women over 40, who may be dealing with the challenges of midlife, weight training can be a powerful tool for improving both physical and mental health.

When starting a weight training program, it is important to work with a qualified trainer or coach who can help to develop a safe and effective program. Women over 40 may have specific health concerns or physical limitations that need to be taken into account when designing a program. A trainer can also provide guidance on proper form and technique, which can help to reduce the risk of injury.

It is also important to remember that weight training is just one part of a healthy lifestyle. Eating a nutritious diet, getting enough sleep, and managing stress are all important factors in maintaining good health as we age.

Overall, weight training can be an excellent way for women over 40 to stay healthy, strong, and vibrant. By incorporating weight training into their exercise routine, women can improve their physical and mental health, and enjoy the many benefits of an active lifestyle.